WHY DO I HURT? Workbook

Neuroscience Education Workbook for Patients with Pain

Adriaan Louw
PT, PhD

The procedures and practices described in this book should be implemented in a manner consistent with professional standards set for the circumstances that apply in each situation. Every effort has been made to confirm accuracy of the information presented and to correctly relate generally accepted practices.

The author, editor and publisher cannot accept responsibility for errors or exclusions or for the outcome of the application of the material presented herein. There is no expressed or implied warranty of this book or information imparted by it.

Designed and published by OPTP.
3800 Annapolis Lane N #165
Minneapolis, MN 55447
800.367.7393 I OPTP.com
Copy edited by OPTP.
All images from Adriaan Louw, unless otherwise noted.

ISBN #978-1-942798-05-7

Index

SCIENTIFIC SUPPORT FOR YOUR WORKBOOK

In each section, you will notice some numbers in the sentences. These numbers refer to scientific articles that support the statements in your book. The details of each article are listed at the back of your book.

The fact that you're reading this workbook tells us something about you. You hurt. We can only imagine what you are experiencing: Countless medical appointments, sleepless nights, and pain all the time, not to mention the constant fatigue and sense of despair.

As a medical community we have failed you. We owe you an apology. This workbook brings together years of research, the personal stories of thousands of patients, and the belief that pain can be treated and people in pain can get back to a meaningful life. Is it easy? No. It takes work, but more importantly, it takes you. It's time to take ownership and control of your pain, and, equipped with the right knowledge and support, you can do just that.

Pain is a normal human experience.[1] Without the ability to experience pain, you would not survive. Living in pain, however, is not normal. Our knowledge of how pain works has increased considerably in the last 25 years.[1-3] When pain lasts longer than expected, we now understand the nervous system and brain are the main contributors.[1,2] This holds true for all pain, regardless of where it is in the body, what label has been attached to you or how long it has been going on. A big reason why pain rates are increasing is the fact that too much focus has been placed on tissues, such as muscles, ligaments and joints.[2,3] However, generally speaking, tissues are healed between three and six months. Pain is far more complex than just tissue issues.

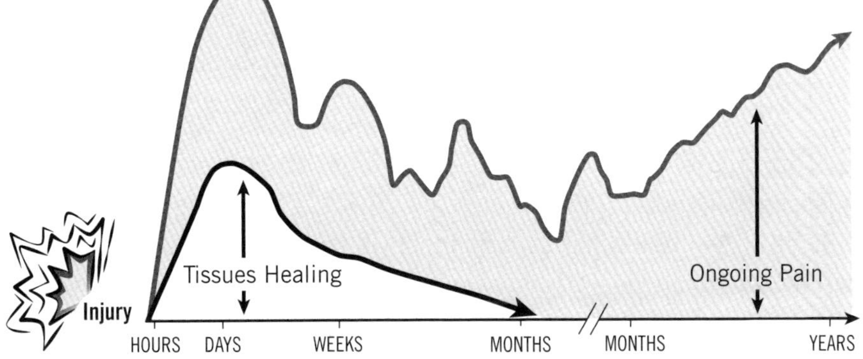

Ongoing pain is more due to sensitive nerves and how the brain processes information from the body and the environment than tissues.[4] This book was written to educate you on how your nerves and brain influence your pain.[5] In most cases people struggling with ongoing pain have more of a "pain problem" than a "tissue problem."[6]

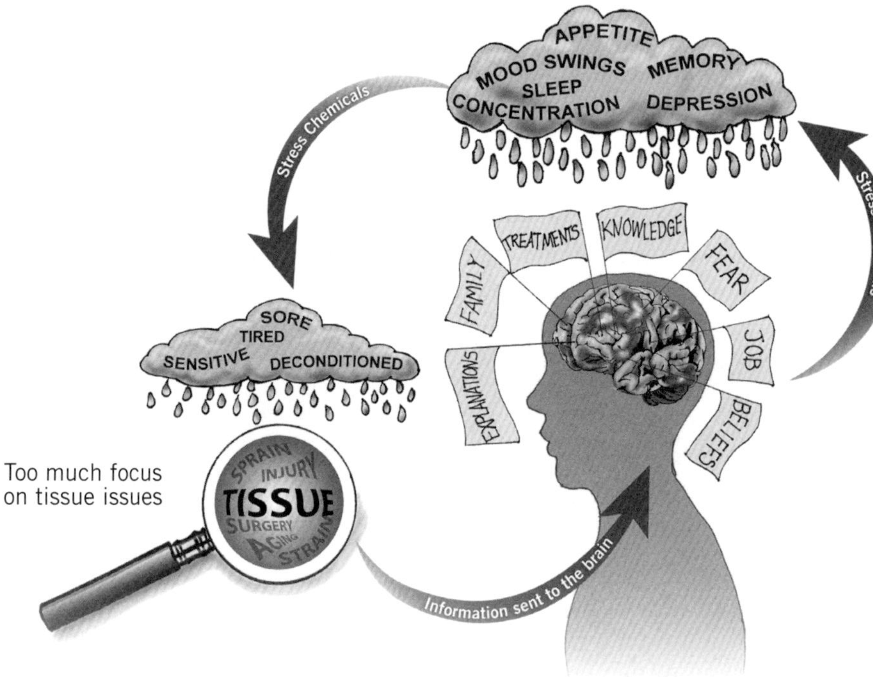

The latest research shows that the more you know about pain and how it works, the better off you'll be.[7,8] This includes moving and functioning better, experiencing less pain, and having an increased ability and interest in doing more healthy exercise and movement. This knowledge is essential in your recovery. Additionally, research has shown that nearly everyone is able to understand the science of the nervous system and pain.[9] So welcome to learning about this science of the nerves and pain, which is more accurately called "the neuroscience of pain."[10]

How to use the workbook

Learning is an active process. We suggest you do one section at a time.[11] Pace yourself. Some of the topics may be emotional, so take your time. Many of our patients experience various emotions, including anger, frustration, low mood, and fatigue when going through this program. This is normal and shows you're paying attention. When asked to, fill in the pages, color where necessary, complete each section's deeper reflection task and discuss this with your closest friends and family, but also reach out to your healthcare provider. You have nothing to lose...except your pain.

SECTION 1: Your personal pain journey

Pain is a personal experience.[3] Everyone's pain experience is unique. Owning your pain involves two key elements. First, don't let anyone, including us, tell you how to feel or what to do about your pain. Become smart about your pain and own your choices. If someone on your healthcare team is not treating you well or not listening to you, feel free to "fire" that person. This is the first step in taking control of your pain. The second important aspect of owning your pain is to realize that the true ability to change your pain starts within you. Our job is to educate, explain, guide and motivate. Ultimately, you need to help...you.

Your story

If you could write your personal pain story, how would it sound? Have you ever heard someone else talk about their pain, only to find yourself nodding along for most of it? Yes, there are common themes when it comes to dealing with pain. Below is a list of common experiences people in pain struggle with. As you go through the list and something sounds familiar, check the box. Not all of them will apply, but look at the bigger picture of failed treatments, various diagnoses and numerous tests.

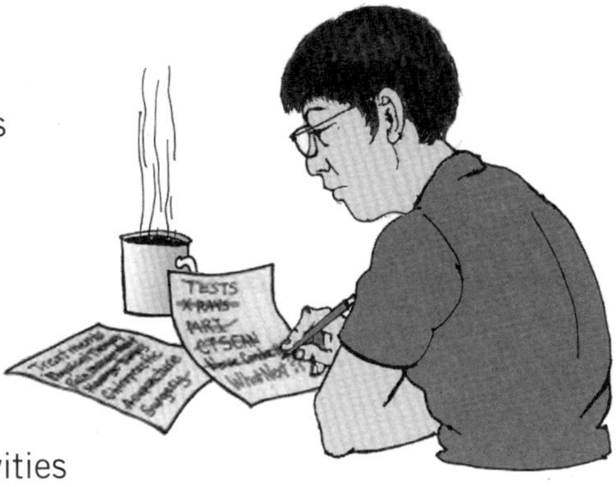

- ☐ You've had pain for several months or years
- ☐ Your pain has spread to other areas
- ☐ You have been given several diagnosis labels
- ☐ You've seen numerous healthcare providers
- ☐ You're having problems sleeping
- ☐ You're always tired
- ☐ You've had many medical tests and scans
- ☐ Your pain has limited your ability to do activities
- ☐ Your pain is steadily getting worse instead of better
- ☐ You experience pain when you move and exercise
- ☐ Your family and friends don't understand your pain
- ☐ Your pain has impacted your job and increased worry about money
- ☐ You get help from each new treatment for a while, but then it stops working
- ☐ You feel you are asked to "prove" you hurt

Your medical tests

If you had to make a list of all the tests you've had, how long would it be? How much did it cost? Did the findings help you or add more stress? Have a look at the list below, and check off the tests you've had for your pain. Note how many of each you have had in the space provided.

- ☐ X-rays______
- ☐ CT/CAT scans______
- ☐ Nerve-conduction tests______
- ☐ MRIs______
- ☐ Blood tests______
- ☐ Myelograms______

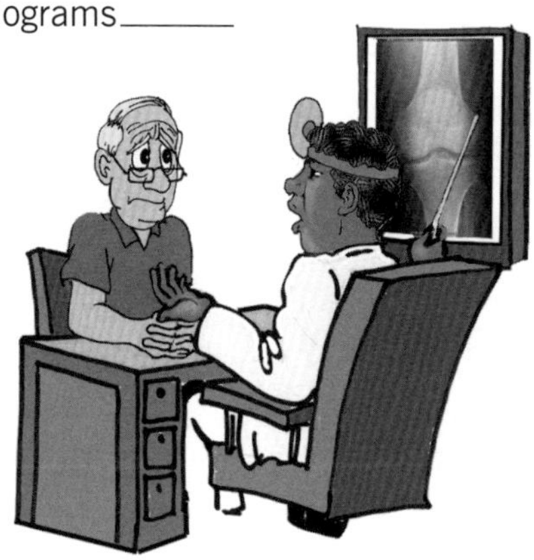

Based on all the tests you've had, one would think you should have some really great information about your worsening pain. Unfortunately, you likely have no new answers as to why you hurt, if the pain will get worse, what you should do for the pain or what can be done for it by your healthcare provider.

Your treatments

How many different types of professionals have you seen? Your list includes most if not all of these professions. Go ahead, mark the ones you've seen.

- ☐ Family Doctor______
- ☐ Pain Management Specialist______
- ☐ Neurologist______
- ☐ Massage Therapist______
- ☐ Psychologist______
- ☐ Nurse Practitioner______
- ☐ Physical Therapist______
- ☐ Orthopedic Surgeon______
- ☐ Chiropractor______
- ☐ Rheumatologist______
- ☐ Physician Assistant______
- ☐ Podiatrist______

If you've had pain for a long time, the list may include your family doctor, five different physical therapists, eight chiropractors, three different pain management specialists and four different massage therapists. Write the numbers next to each category above to show how many of each you've seen. Adding to the frustration, if any of these well-meaning people and their treatments helped, it only helped for a while before the pain increased or returned.

Your medical expenses

How much money have you spent trying to get help for your pain? This may include co-pays for medical visits, pillows, mattresses, lotions, vitamins, shoes, inserts, medicine and more. Everyone has a magic cure, and it comes at a price. By now you may have spent a lot of money and yet, you're not any closer to having less pain. If anything, the pain is getting worse.

Your drugs

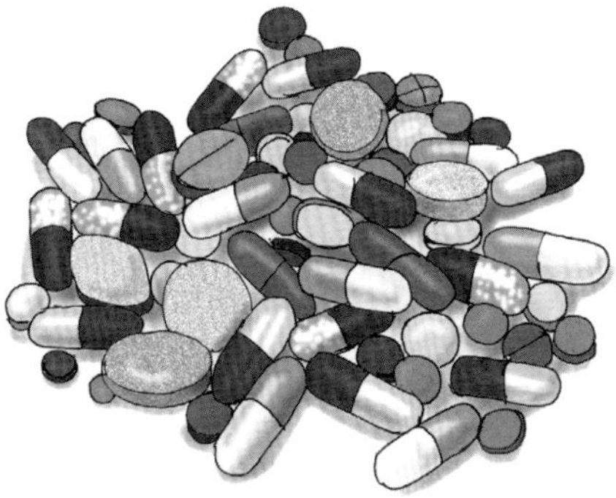

The mainstay treatment you have received is probably big doses of various drugs. Depending on how long you've had pain, you could have gone through various forms of pain medication, muscle relaxants, antidepressants and the now popular membrane stabilizing drugs such as Cymbalta™, Neurontin™ or Lyrica™. Skillful delivery of medication is only a small part of a bigger treatment plan that will be discussed throughout your workbook. Unfortunately, these medications sometimes cause more symptoms than the pain itself with undesirable side effects such as fatigue, drowsiness, soreness, stomach irritation and more. The purpose of this section is not to tell you that you should or should not take medication. That is your physician's job. The purpose is to highlight the experience of the typical patient struggling with pain.

Your perspective

As you reflect on your personal pain story, does any of this sound familiar? What advice would you give to someone struggling with pain? What do you know about your pain? Here is a list given to us by a patient struggling with years of pain. Go ahead, look at it and, if any of it sounds familiar, check the boxes:

- ☐ I don't want it.
- ☐ No one believes me.
- ☐ It's not getting better.
- ☐ Nothing helps me.
- ☐ The future looks bleak.
- ☐ I'll have to learn to live with it.

Any others you'd like to add? ______________________________

____

____

As you look at all the issues you have been dealing with and live with every day, how does that make you feel? This is a good time to take inventory of your personal situation. Here is a personal pain inventory. Go ahead and rate the different areas of your life right now, zero indicating not good at all and 10 being really good.

	NOT GOOD					AVERAGE					REALLY GOOD
Overall Mood	0	1	2	3	4	5	6	7	8	9	10
Sleeping Enough	0	1	2	3	4	5	6	7	8	9	10
Eating Healthy	0	1	2	3	4	5	6	7	8	9	10
Exercising Regularly	0	1	2	3	4	5	6	7	8	9	10
Getting Daily Tasks Done	0	1	2	3	4	5	6	7	8	9	10
Stress Level	0	1	2	3	4	5	6	7	8	9	10
Personal Time	0	1	2	3	4	5	6	7	8	9	10
Motivated and Have Goals	0	1	2	3	4	5	6	7	8	9	10
Family Relationships	0	1	2	3	4	5	6	7	8	9	10
Work Situation	0	1	2	3	4	5	6	7	8	9	10
	NOT GOOD					AVERAGE					REALLY GOOD

Your journey

With all of these experiences and the apparent inability of the medical system to help, you likely feel trapped, like you're going through the motions, or even worse, stuck in a roundabout.[12] Yes, the average American can have major issues with roundabouts, which should be a book all by itself! Once you experience an injury, accident, undergo surgery or a lot of emotional stress, it is normal to experience pain. Pain grabs your attention and makes you do something about it. Unfortunately, all of the tests, treatments, experiences, frustration and information you have undergone pushed you toward the roundabout. This has led to a feeling of helplessness, increased worries associated with your pain and decreased movement and activity. Where are you in the roundabout right now? How many times have you been around the roundabout?

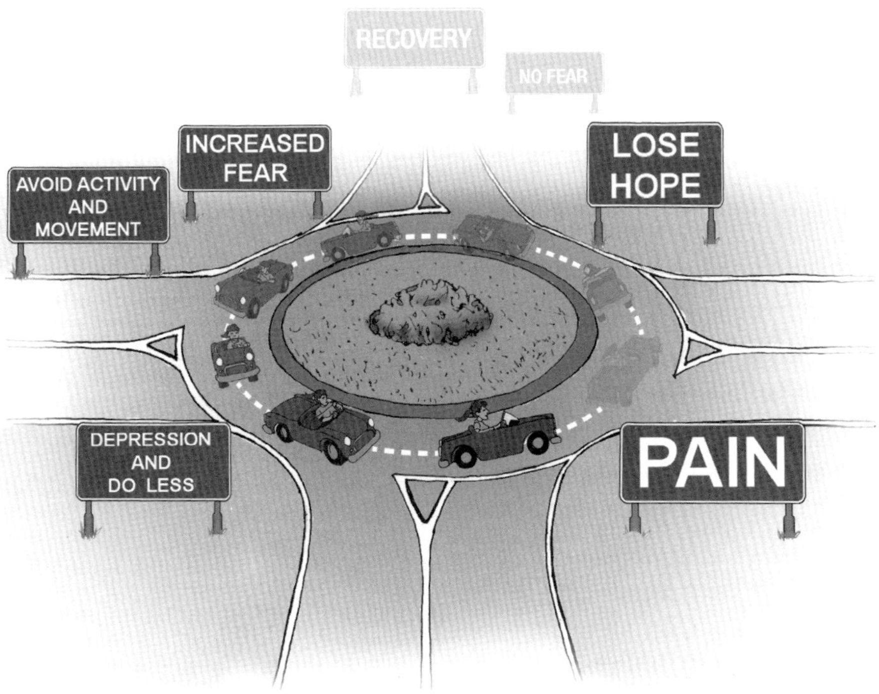

TASK 1

After examining your personal pain journey, do you see yourself as being stuck in the pain roundabout?
What do you think are the key factors keeping you there?
What is your initial reaction to the idea that there is a difference between a tissue problem and a pain problem?

2

SECTION 2: Your body's alarm system

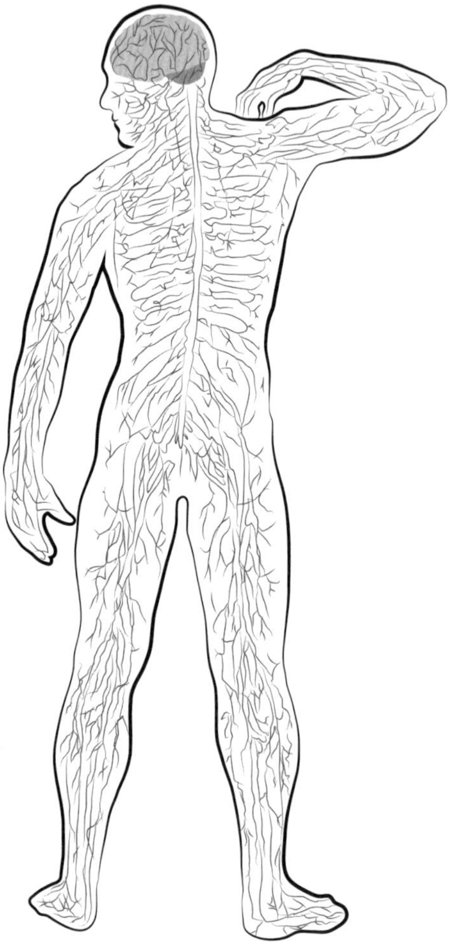

If you were to step on a rusted nail with your bare foot, would you want to know about it?[11] Yes, of course! Why? So you DO SOMETHING about it, such as taking the nail out, bandaging the foot and getting a tetanus shot. How do you know there's a nail in your foot? Do you have eyeballs at the bottom of your foot? Of course not! Then how do we know about the nail?

Our body has a very sophisticated alarm system that tells us when we have an injury, accident, surgery or even emotional stress.[1,5] This alarm system is called the nervous system. The human body contains 45 miles of nerves and more than 400 individual nerves, all connected like a network of roads. These nerves connect all body parts to the spinal cord so messages can be sent from your tissues to the brain for analysis. Your nerves monitor your body and inform you and your brain of anything going on in your body.[13]

At any given time, nerves have a little bit of electricity running through them. This is normal and shows you're alive.

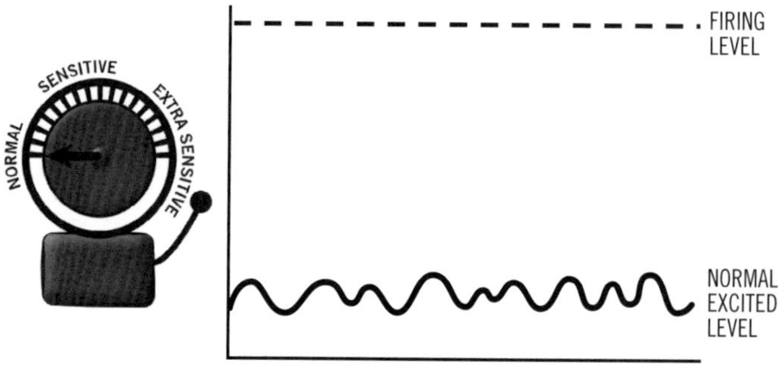

When you step on the nail, your alarm system goes off, firing a danger message to the brain. This in turn produces pain. The pain makes you stop, take care of the issue and, eventually, you get on with your life. The alarm system steadily calms down to its original resting level ready to fire again if needed. Brilliant system!

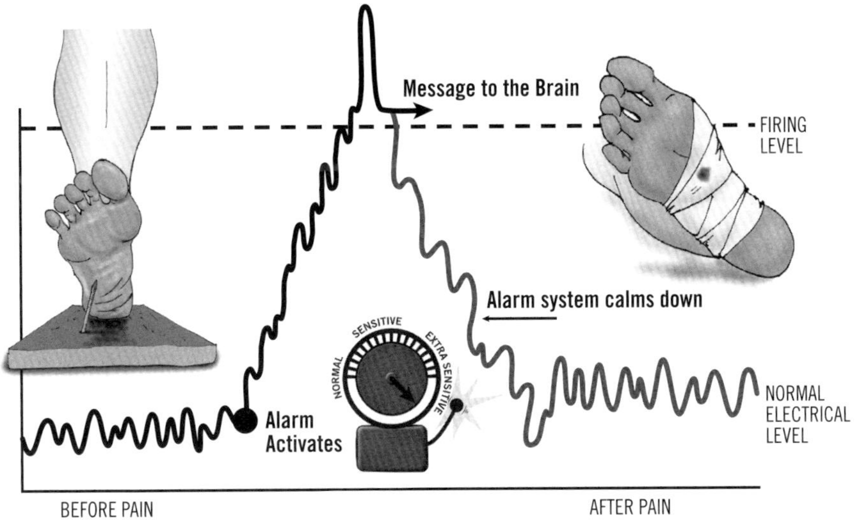

Your trigger

When a threat is present it may set off the alarm. Threats come in a variety of forms and the main ones are listed below.[1] Go ahead, review them and mark the ones that you have experienced.

- ☐ Injury
- ☐ Accident
- ☐ Fracture
- ☐ Surgery
- ☐ Sprain
- ☐ Age changes in tissues
- ☐ Emotional stress
- ☐ Bracing or casts
- ☐ Illness

Your alarm system's response

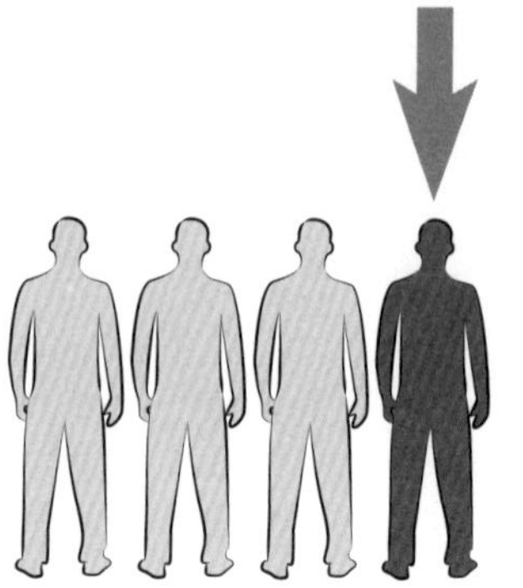

One or several of the stressors triggered your alarm system. Once your alarm system activated, you went for help; you may have gone to the emergency room, seen your family doctor, had an X-ray, etc. Once you sought out help and received treatment, the alarm system should have calmed down. However, our growing pain research now shows that with one in four people in this world, something triggers their alarm system, but the alarm never fully calms all the way back down.[14] This leaves an extra-sensitive alarm system.

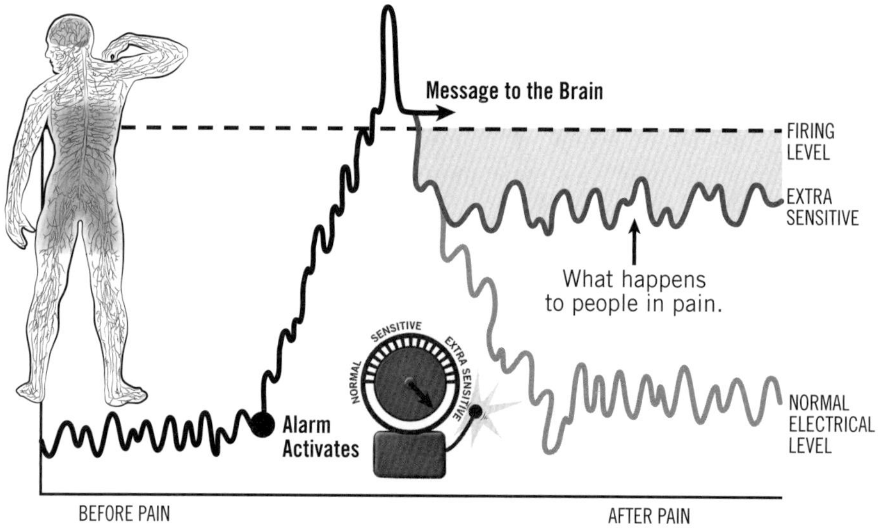

Look at the next two drawings. Before you developed pain, you were able to perform any task quite easily and for long periods, such as driving, doing dishes, or working on a computer. But since you developed pain, you've noticed and reported it doesn't take but a few minutes of the same task to experience pain. No wonder you think something must be wrong! The main issue is an extra-sensitive alarm system.[11]

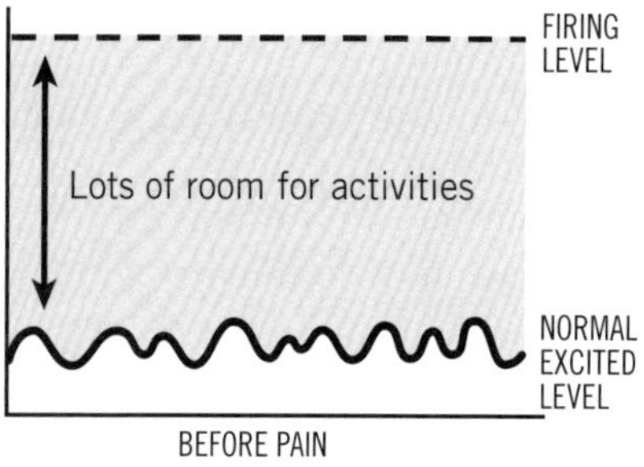

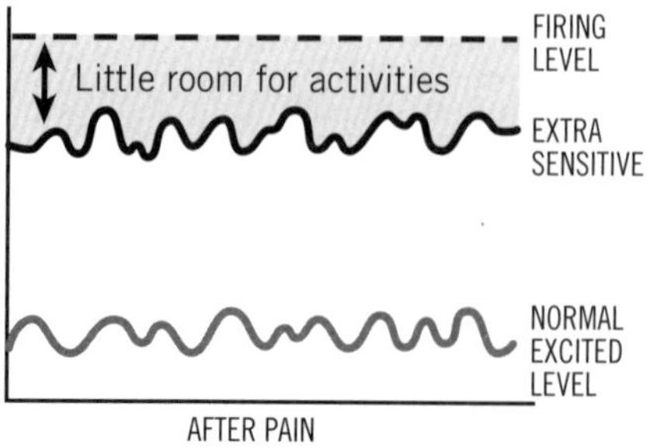

How has your extra-sensitive alarm system changed your life?

Use the tables below and write down five things you used to be able to do, but now struggle to do, or have given up doing. Indicate how the activities are different before and after your pain.

BEFORE PAIN	AFTER PAIN

A key message for you is that tissues heal and a large part of why you still hurt is due to an extra-sensitive alarm system. As long as medical tests and treatments assume the answers are in your tissues (joints, muscles, etc.), it is unlikely you will get better. We must step back and look in the right place: Your nervous system.

TASK 2

Look at the activities you used to be able to do before your alarm system became extra sensitive. How do you feel about the impact this has made on your life?

It is okay to feel anger or even grief about your losses. But, if you get stuck there, you are unlikely to find an exit from the roundabout.

Finally, look at the list again and reflect. How much of what you're experiencing is more due to an extra-sensitive alarm system versus a tissue issue?

SECTION 3: Knowing your alarm system has become extra sensitive

In all the years we have used the extra-sensitive alarm system story to help people understand more about their pain, three very important questions are usually asked.[11]

1. **How do you know that my nerves are extra sensitive? None of my tests reported this.**
2. **Why didn't my nerves calm down? My neighbor had a similar injury and she's fine.**
3. **How can the alarm system be turned down?**

The last question is likely THE right question to ask and we cannot wait to answer that one. We do, however, need to cover the first two questions. They are essential for you to develop increased knowledge of pain and how pain works. So, how do we know your alarm system is extra sensitive?

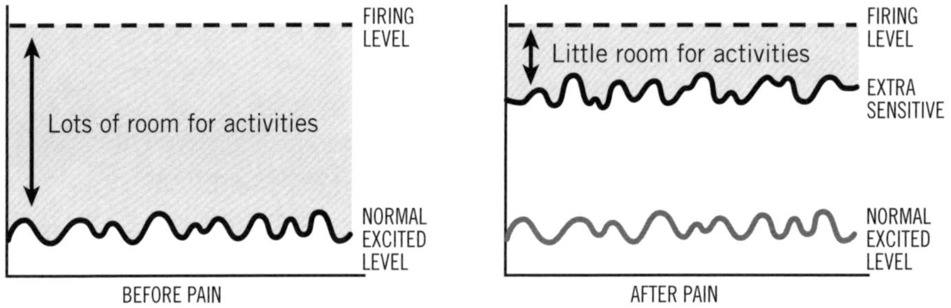

You told us

The easy answer is that you have already told us. If you look at all the things you used to be able to do before developing pain and how this has changed, it's an indication of how the extra-sensitive alarm system has limited your activity.

Your doctor told us

No, your doctor did not call us behind your back. But, if we look at the list of medications you've been taking (antidepressants, membrane stabilizers and muscle relaxants), it is clear your doctor is trying different medications designed to calm your nerves down.

Your examination told us

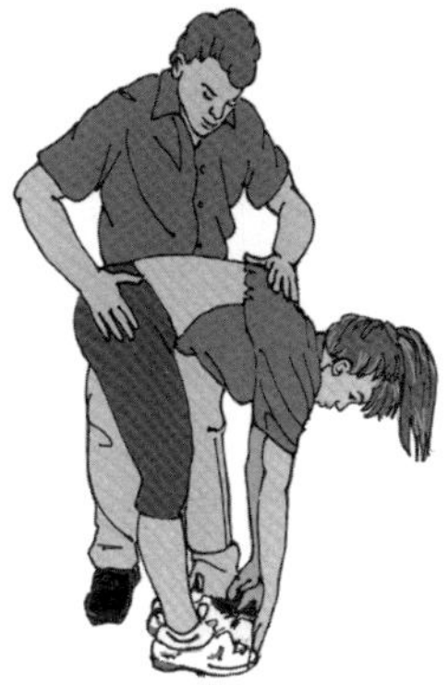

You may also have noticed when your physical therapist examined you with movement tests or touch, you were more sensitive than usual, especially around the areas you're experiencing pain.

Your nerve sensors told us

You may have noticed that beyond the "normal" sensitivity described, you have become sensitive to other things, such as cold temperatures, stress and anxiety.[6] You may even feel more pain when you have the flu. This is normal and can easily be explained. Inside your nerves, there are various sensors designed to protect and inform you of any changes in your life and daily environment. Scientists recently identified these sensors and realize there are many different kinds. As we describe these sensors, go ahead and place a checkmark by the ones you think may be part of your pain experience:

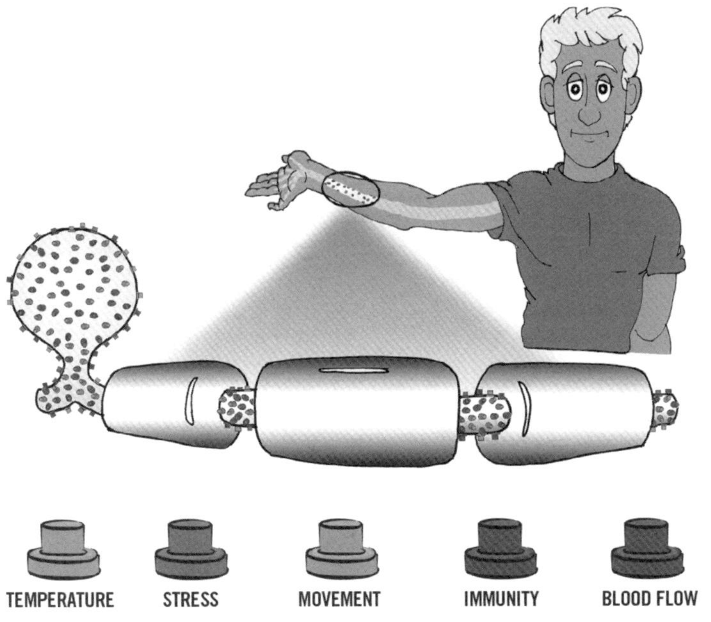

☐ **TEMPERATURE:** There are sensors in nerves that tell you if there is a change in temperature. It's not uncommon to become sensitive to cold temperature and feel more aches and pains in the affected area when it gets cold out.

☐ **STRESS:** There are sensors in nerves that are sensitive to stress chemicals flowing in your blood. The more stressed, anxious, nervous or upset you are, the more you will experience a few more aches and pains, and the more likely additional stress sensors will be activated.

☐ **MOVEMENT:** There are sensors in your nerves which are sensitive to movement and pressure around them. For example, movement after injury may activate a few more sensors and make the movement more sensitive for a little while.

☐ **IMMUNITY:** When you're sick with the flu, there are many immune molecules floating through your body helping you deal with the illness. This is the same following injury or surgery. Recent research shows that when you are really worried or have an inflamed body part, you'll have an immune response. Nerves have sensors telling them about the increased immune molecules, and the immune chemicals produced can make you ache.

☐ **BLOOD FLOW:** There are sensors in your nerves that are sensitive to the amount of blood around your tissues. When blood flow slows down slightly, for example after sitting too long, these sensors "wake up" and make the nerves sensitive.

KEY POINTS ABOUT NERVE SENSORS:

✔ **When you developed pain, your nerves increased their sensitivity to protect you**

✔ **This is a normal response and happens in every human being**

✔ **These sensors are constantly updated based on your environment and can shift for the better!**

Your neighbors told us

Don't worry, your neighbors did not call us, but your body parts have neighbors and they can tell us about your extra-sensitive alarm system as well. When you develop pain in an area of your body and the nerves in that area "wake up," there are usually some interested neighbors.[5,11] Think of it this way: If the alarm in your house goes off in the middle of the night, it probably wakes up your next door neighbors. They are curious and concerned about you. If the alarm keeps going, some neighbors down the street may also wake up.

Nerves work the same way. The areas where you are experiencing pain have the alarm system going off all the time, and the tissue's neighbors have been awakened. It is not uncommon to experience some sensitivity, such as aches and pains in areas adjacent to the involved areas, or to sense a spreading pain. Spreading pain is not necessarily associated with more injury or tissue issues, but more likely irritated neighbors.

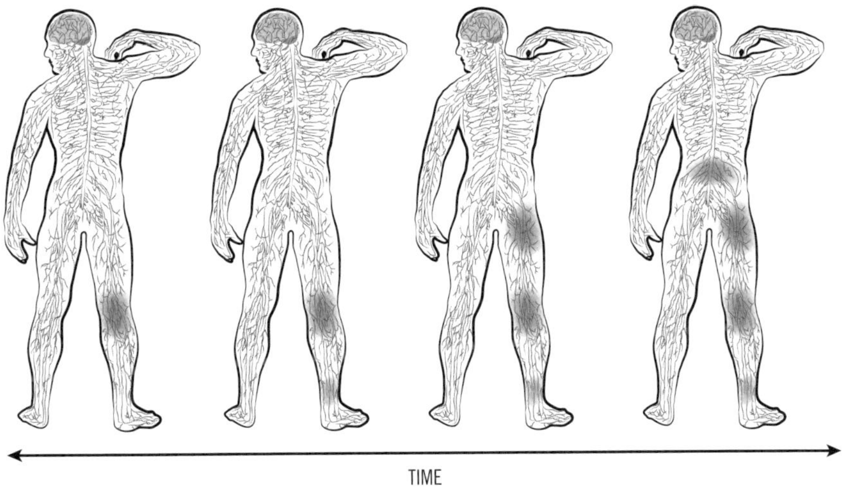

As you can see, many of the issues you are dealing with can be explained. The best part, as you will see later, is that the more you understand this new information about pain, the better off you will be. While you're in the pain roundabout it's hard to see the light at the end of the tunnel. All of these processes we have described can be changed for the better, so keep going, work through the book and you will see how.

TASK 3

As you reflect on the changes in your activities, the medications you take, your responses when examined by healthcare practitioners, your sensitivity to things like cold and stress, and your "neighbors," do you now believe you have more of a pain issue versus a tissue issue? Which of these clues stands out to you the most? How do you feel about the fact that there is a good explanation for all of these symptoms that have been so disruptive to your life?

SECTION 4: Why did this happen to you?

In some people, there are so many issues surrounding pain that the brain decides it's logical to keep the alarm system elevated. Injuries, accidents and surgery do not occur in a vacuum, but rather, they are strongly influenced by other factors at home, work, and throughout your medical journey.[15] Many studies have shown that our home life and work environment play a big role in either increasing or decreasing our pain. The following are some issues that keep the alarm system sensitive. Yes, go ahead and mark the ones you have experienced.

☐ **FAILED TREATMENT**

Perhaps, by this point, you have experienced failed treatment. This is unfortunate and certainly not helpful. When you take medication, or receive physical therapy, chiropractic treatments or injections that don't work, the brain's worry increases. "Why is the treatment not working? Why did the injections help my neighbor, but not me?" As long as your brain asks these questions, your alarm system will remain elevated.

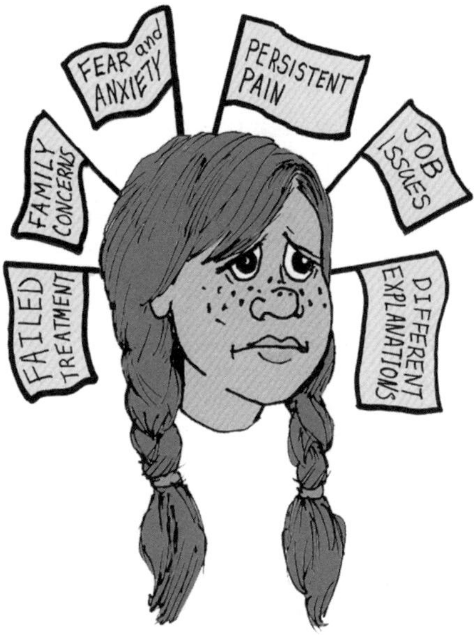

☐ **DIFFERENT EXPLANATIONS FOR YOUR PAIN**

From the time you developed pain, you've probably heard many opinions. It's common to seek answers, but unfortunately when you get different explanations for your pain from various people, it confuses your brain. You begin to think there are several different things that are falling apart. This provides little incentive for the brain to turn down the alarm system. Thoughts such as the following add stress: "This must be bad since no one can find the problem" or, "The problem must be super-complex since no one can agree on what's happening."

☐ **FAMILY AND JOB**

Since your pain started, your family life and your job have been hijacked. This includes endless doctor and therapy visits, expensive tests, lost work time, frustration, concerns about being able to do your job, concerns about the future and money issues. These thoughts add more concern for the brain and, once again, provide little incentive to turn the alarm system down.

□ **FEAR**

Considering the failed treatments, job and family issues and various explanations for your pain, there is going to be a lot of uncertainty. The uncertainty is usually accompanied by anxiety or fear. These reactions are quite common. Unfortunately, it has been shown that fear of injury or re-injury, and even fear of exercise or movement, can keep your alarm system turned on.

The list of issues that can keep an alarm system extra sensitive is long and personal. This is again why pain is such an individual experience. In people like you, struggling with ongoing pain, the alarm system is extra sensitive and many issues, other than the health of your tissues, are keeping the alarm system elevated.

Can you identify a few things in your life that have caused your alarm system to remain extra sensitive? Fill them in on the picture below. We call these yellow (danger) flags, which add threat. You may even want to add more flags.

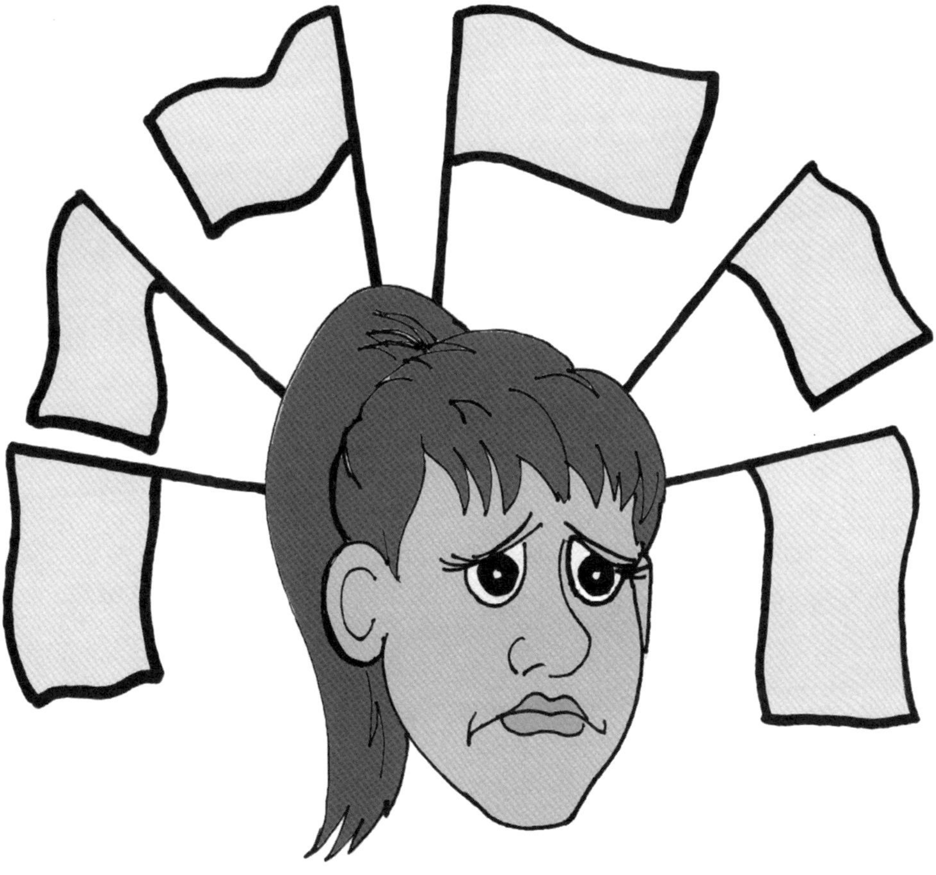

Yes, but…I have "issues in my tissues"

We are getting closer to the all-important third question: How do I turn down an extra-sensitive alarm system? Before we get to this exciting part of your workbook, we need to address a very important issue: Your tissues. In the last 300 years, in order to help people in pain, the vast majority of the medical system has focused on tissue issues. How is this working out for us? Pain rates have almost doubled in the last 30 years and it is now estimated that one in four people in this world struggle with some form of persistent pain. The use of prescription pain medication has increased dramatically, yet pain is at an all-time high. Even worse, pain medications have been shown to help very little, often increasing pain and having serious side effects and consequences. Why is pain not getting better? There are many factors, but our scientific team believes it is healthcare's over-emphasis on seeking answers in the tissues alone.

- **There are many people who have injured, aged or deconditioned tissues, yet experience little to no pain[2]**
- **On the flip side, there are many people who experience significant pain, yet their scans and medical tests show little or no damage in the tissues**

Consider these statistics:

Neck

- Among people with significant "arthritic changes" in their neck scans, only 10% actually have neck pain[16]
- In demolition derby drivers who crash 1500 times during their career, only 2% experience long-lasting neck pain[17]

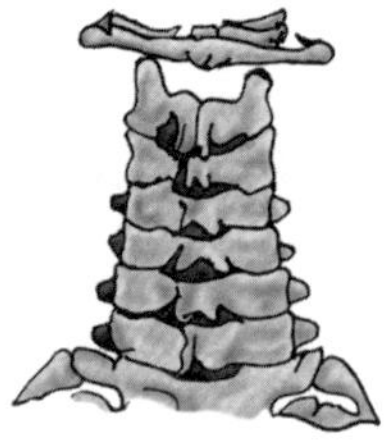

Shoulder

- Among people who have had successful surgery, experience no pain and regain all movement, 1 in 5 still have a muscle tear[18]
- In people over age 30 who have a shoulder muscle tear, only 1 in 3 actually experience pain or limited activity[19]

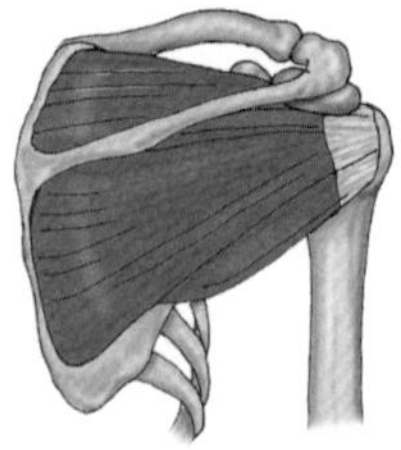

Low Back

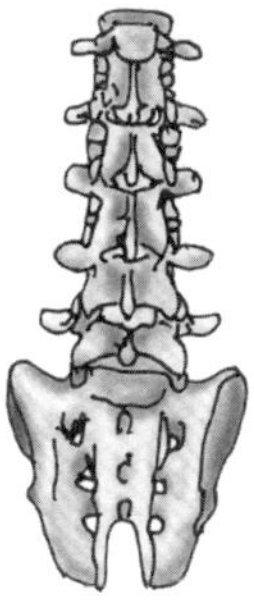

- Among people with no back pain, more than 40% have a bulging disc on their scan; bulging discs reabsorb over time.[20]
- In older patients, scans often show "wrinkles on the inside (arthritis)," yet most people seeking help with back pain are middle-aged[21]

Hip

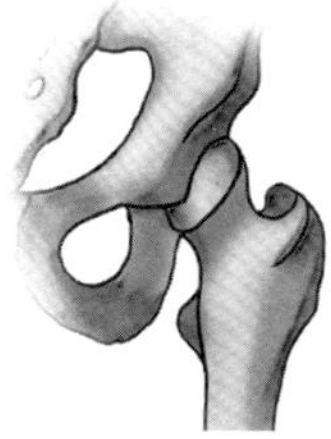

- Among people with no hip pain, 75% of their scans still show tissue issues[22]
- In hockey players with no hip pain, 2 out of 3 have scans that show significant arthritis to their hips[23]

Knee

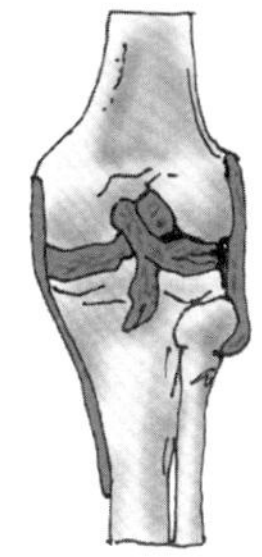

- Among people with arthritis on their knee scan, only 50% experience pain[24]
- Among college basketball players with significant issues on their knee scans, 1 in 3 have no knee pain.[25]

Tissue issues can and do result in pain. And yes, treatments may help tissues. But the overall message is that pain is far more complex than just tissues, **especially ongoing pain**.[2] Treating pain needs a large-scale, broad approach.

TASK 4

Non-tissue issues such as failed treatment, fear, family and finances, were discussed as contributors to the pain experience. Do you agree that these outside factors can drive the sensitivity of the alarm system up? As you filled in your flags, which ones do you think pose the biggest threat and keep you circling through the roundabout? What is your reaction to the statistics that illustrate injured tissue doesn't have to hurt? Do you find yourself wanting to hold on to your "tissue issue explanations" despite this knowledge? Many people feel reluctant to let that go, but accepting that ongoing pain is a multi-factorial, complex issue is key to getting on the road to recovery.

SECTION 5: Your brain meetings

Yes, we know...we promised you we will teach you how to turn the alarm system down. There are, however, two important, must-discuss issues about your pain we need to show you before we conquer the all-important treatment strategy: Pain meetings and lions. To help you understand your pain, and more importantly what pain has done to you, we need to teach you how your brain gets hijacked by pain. This is normal, but all of these changes make the pain struggle even more difficult.

For years it was generally believed that there is a single pain area in the brain. When you stub your toe, the light bulb flashes and there it is; pain. If pain were that simple, it would be easy to cut this area out of the brain, and all pain would be gone. When you have a pain experience, it is now well established by brain scans that different areas of your brain are involved in processing the experience.[3,26] We think of this as your brain having a "pain meeting." Areas of the brain that usually perform other tasks are used to process pain, which affects how they perform their normal tasks.

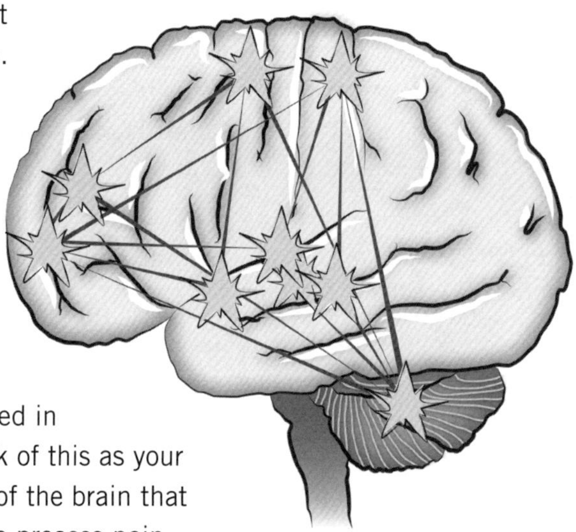

Look at the list below and see if you are experiencing any of the issues we commonly see in people with ongoing pain. Not all will apply, but go ahead and place checkmarks next to the ones that you have experienced.

- ☐ Your muscles are tired and sore
- ☐ You have problems remembering things
- ☐ You notice food tastes different
- ☐ You notice similar pain on your other side
- ☐ You get mentally tired
- ☐ You are more anxious and nervous
- ☐ You're not very motivated
- ☐ You move differently
- ☐ You get "hot flashes"
- ☐ You focus a lot on your pain
- ☐ You have problems focusing and concentrating
- ☐ You have problems staying on task
- ☐ You tend to eat more than usual
- ☐ Your pain seems to be spreading

If you look at the list we gave you, it corresponds to areas in the brain we now know are part of the pain meeting. When pain uses these areas, the original task allocated to that area suffers. For example, when you experience pain, the memory area is called to the pain meeting and...memory suffers, especially short-term memory. Is there something wrong with your brain? No, it's just trying to deal with your pain and all the issues surrounding it... doctor's visits, medical bills, failed treatments, job stress, etc. If you look at the list below, you will see which areas of your brain are in the pain meeting. As you review the list, check off the ones that apply.

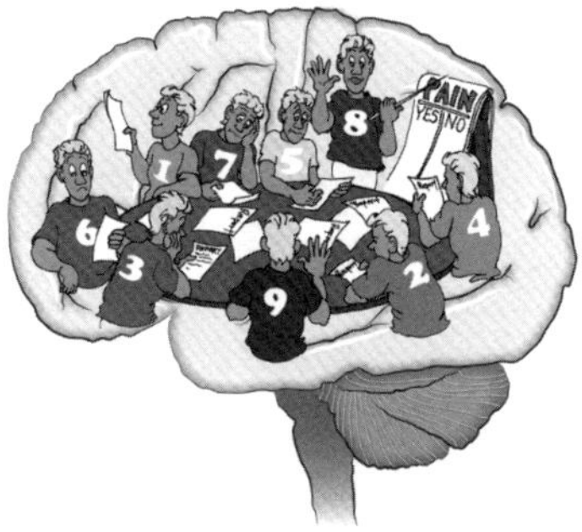

☐ 1. MUSCLES
With the brain having a pain meeting, muscles struggle to do their job, leaving some of them overworked and sore.

☐ 2. FOCUS
Being involved in a pain meeting causes us to become mentally tired and have trouble with focus and concentration.

☐ 3. PROBLEM SOLVING
Staying on task as well as keeping appointments and numbers straight is tough when we're preoccupied with a pain meeting.

☐ 4. FEAR
We experience increased fear of movement and pain when we're busy attending a pain meeting.

☐ 5. BODY MAPS
Because we're in a pain meeting and are extra busy multi-tasking, pain spreads in the body and is felt in adjacent areas.

☐ 6. STRESS RESPONSES
We often have problems regulating stress chemicals, body temperature or eating when forced to attend a pain meeting.

☐ 7. MEMORY
Because we're preoccupied with our pain meeting, we often have problems remembering things, especially in the short-term.

☐ 8. MOTIVATION
Our motivation sometimes decreases due to attending a pain meeting, causing us to become tired and fatigued.

☐ 9. TISSUE ISSUES
Another disadvantage of being held up in a pain meeting is that we aren't able to correctly analyze messages from the tissues.

A common but unfortunate saying is that pain is in your head. That saying implies that pain is not real; it's fabricated. This is not true. Your brain **does** play a big role in your pain experience, so technically yes, pain involves the brain, and your brain happens to be located in your head. But this is an issue of how the brain processes information, not an issue of the imagination!

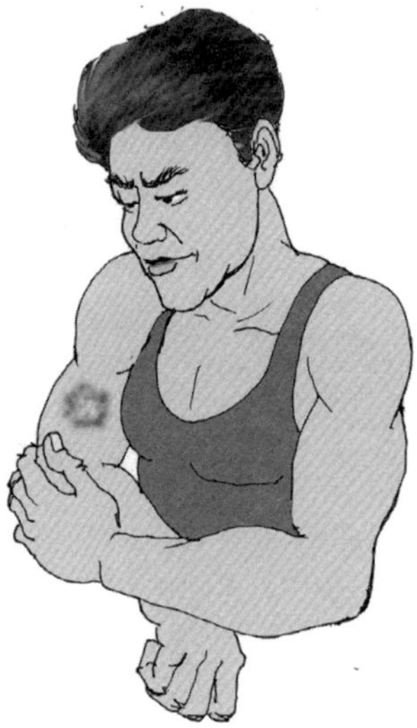

Have you ever seen a bruise on your body and had no idea where it came from? Here is an example of an injury and no pain. If you experienced pain, you'd know the exact date and time. The brain has to be part of the pain experience. In this case the brain decided to shut the danger messages down, and you kept going with what you were doing and pain was not experienced. Who made this decision? Your brain!

The best part? As you learn about pain, your brain gets smarter and over time puts an end to these pain meetings. All of the issues you marked on your list, just as they have become worse over time, can also get better over time.

TASK 5

As you look at the areas you marked on your list as being stuck in a pain meeting and unable to focus on their usual job, which ones have alarmed you the most? How do you feel about the possibility of your brain putting an end to these pain meetings so the various areas of your brain can get back to doing their respective jobs 100%?

SECTION 6: Your lion

If a big, roaring African lion jumped into your room right now, what would you do? Take a nap? Focus on your posture or conserve energy? Here are some specific questions. Go ahead, answer them.

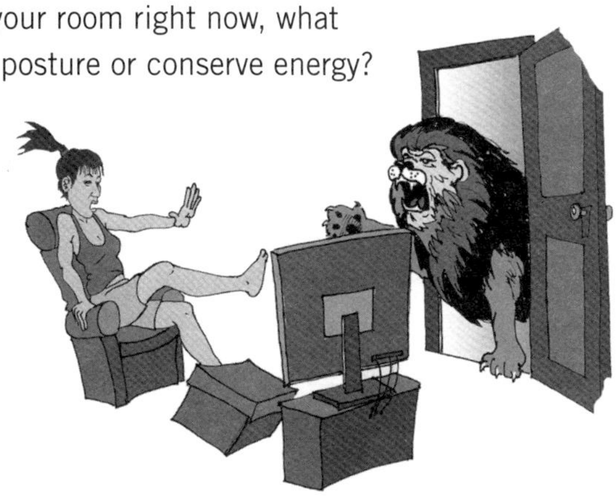

A lion has jumped into the room!

- Is your heart rate up or down? Why?
- Is it time for a nap? Why or why not?
- Is your posture important right now?
- Which muscles are important to use?
- If you have food in your belly, do you want to spend time digesting it?
- Are you interested in sex at this time? (If you are, you have some serious issues...)
- Are you wanting to store energy for winter?

The short and easy answer is that our body produces stress chemicals that cause some body systems to ramp up and other body systems to slow down or stop, for the time being, while we deal with the lion in the room. Now, when the local zookeeper comes and removes the lion, all the systems calm down, return to normal and you sink into your seat. This "fight and flight" system is a normal response in all people facing stress in their life.[6,27]

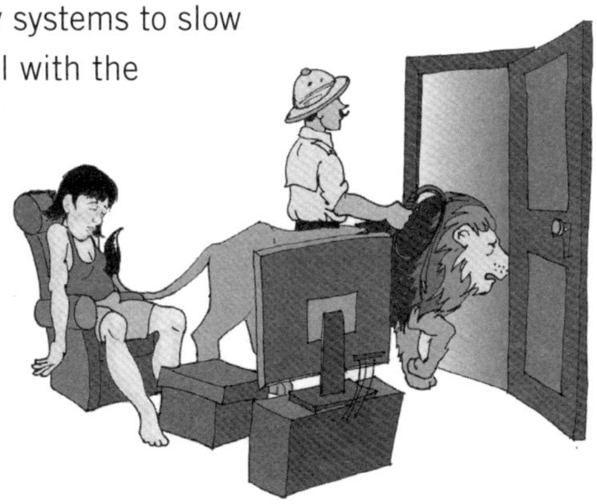

In line with everything you have been dealing with, look at the following list. If any of these apply to you and your pain experience, check them off.

- ☐ Ongoing pain
- ☐ Exercise and movement hurt
- ☐ Fatigue
- ☐ No one wants to help
- ☐ No hope for the future
- ☐ Constant pain
- ☐ Job and money issues
- ☐ Different explanations for pain
- ☐ Family issues
- ☐ Constant stress
- ☐ Failed treatment
- ☐ Life is miserable
- ☐ There is no hope
- ☐ Have to prove you hurt
- ☐ Told to "live with it"

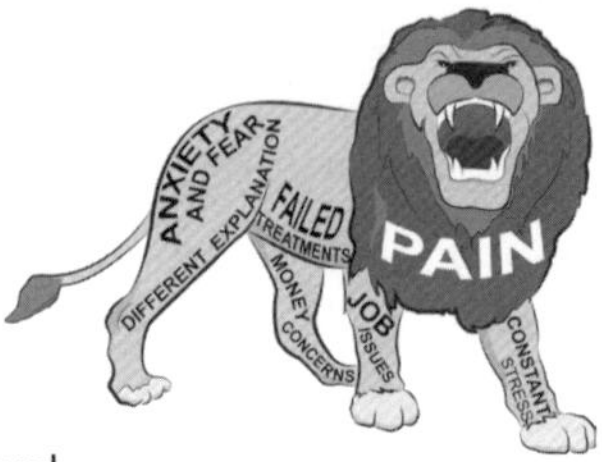

What does the lion story have to do with you? Everything in your life associated with the struggle of pain is bundled together and represents a lion or a constant threat in your life. From the moment you wake, the lion is there and it follows you around all day long, week after week, month after month and year after year. How long has your lion been around? Go ahead, take the issues you marked on the list and "fill in" your lion below.

Our stress systems are designed to act quickly and aggressively, and then to turn off. If they stay turned on for months and years, what happens? You run out of steam, you get tired. Some muscles become tight and tender, while other muscles become tired. You have trouble falling asleep or getting restful sleep. Many of the changes you're experiencing are a consequence of "the lion" being in your life. It's time to make your lion smaller.

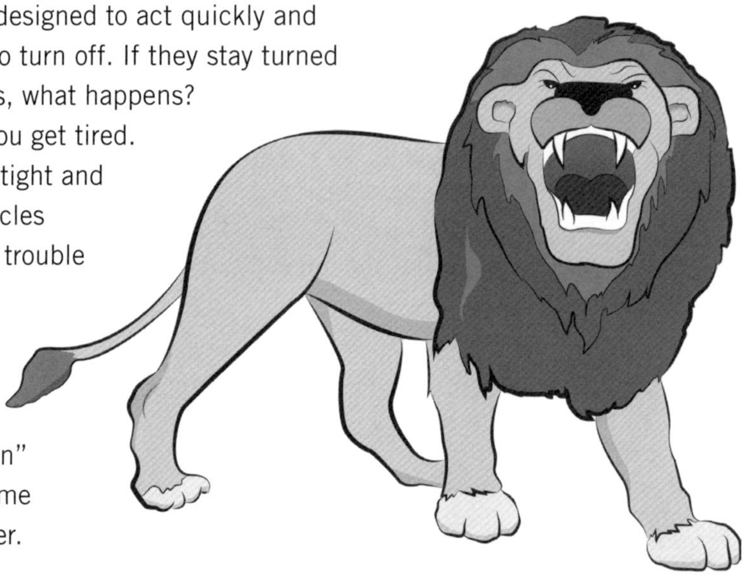

TASK 6

Look at the picture of the lion you filled in. Look at the words. As you imagine your lion shrinking down to a cute lion cub, which words would you like to see disappear first? What action steps might make erasing those words possible?

All of the strategies we will be discussing to help turn down your extra-sensitive alarm system also help with so many of these other issues you're facing. So, back to the all-important question: How do we turn down an extra-sensitive alarm system?[11]

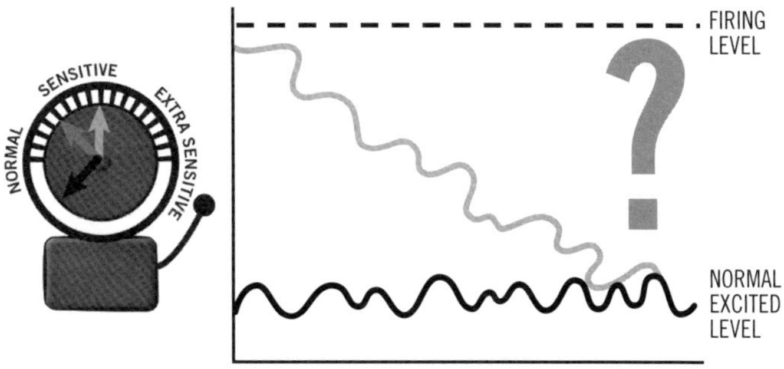

To understand what we mean by "turning the alarm system down," we need to teach you about your brain's pharmacy. The pain you experience is affected by very powerful medicine in the brain. Although many people can name several pain medications you can buy over the counter, few know the powerful pain medicine your brain produces. The world's most sophisticated and powerful pharmacy is situated in your brain. The brain uses chemicals, such as endorphins, enkephalins, opioids and serotonin, to help us ease pain.[1]

WET BRAIN

A wet brain is the description of a brain with a faucet, turned open and flushing pain medication down the spinal cord to dampen incoming danger messages. When you stub your toe, you may experience severe pain for a short while. The toe hurts much less within a few seconds. In this case, the brain uses endorphins and other chemicals to ease the pain experience. These drugs are also important in survival situations and during incidents where people have big injuries, yet experience little to no pain. Can you recall a story where someone had a significant injury, yet experienced little pain? Write it down:

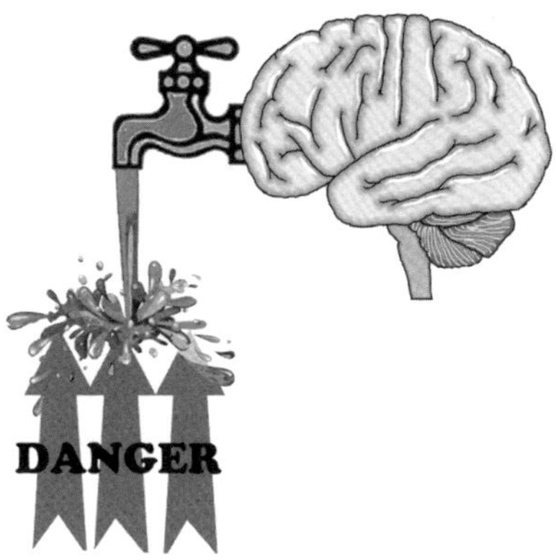

____

____

____

____

DRY BRAIN

A dry brain is the opposite. In this scenario, the faucet is closed. The longer you experience pain, the less pain medication the brain produces. Although it seems contrary, it is also a survival strategy by your brain. Remember that your brain is getting more worried about your pain. Because of this, it makes sense to the brain to dry up or close the tap and stop the medicine from altering the pain experience so you know exactly what is going on.

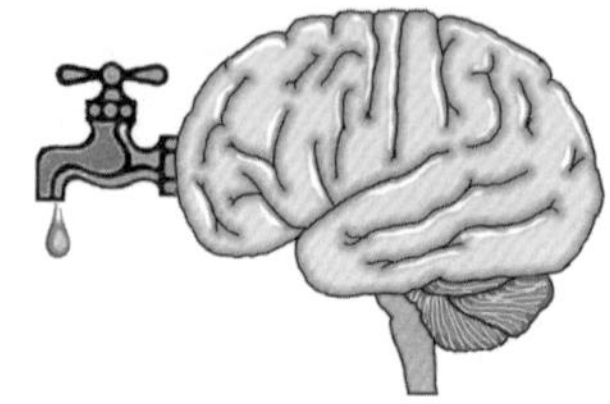

The four pillars:

In order to turn down your alarm system (and pain), we need to get the brain to produce more pain medication. Research has shown there are many ways to help the brain start making more pain medication without the use of drugs. In particular, extensive research has shown there are four key strategies that MUST be in place in order to recover:

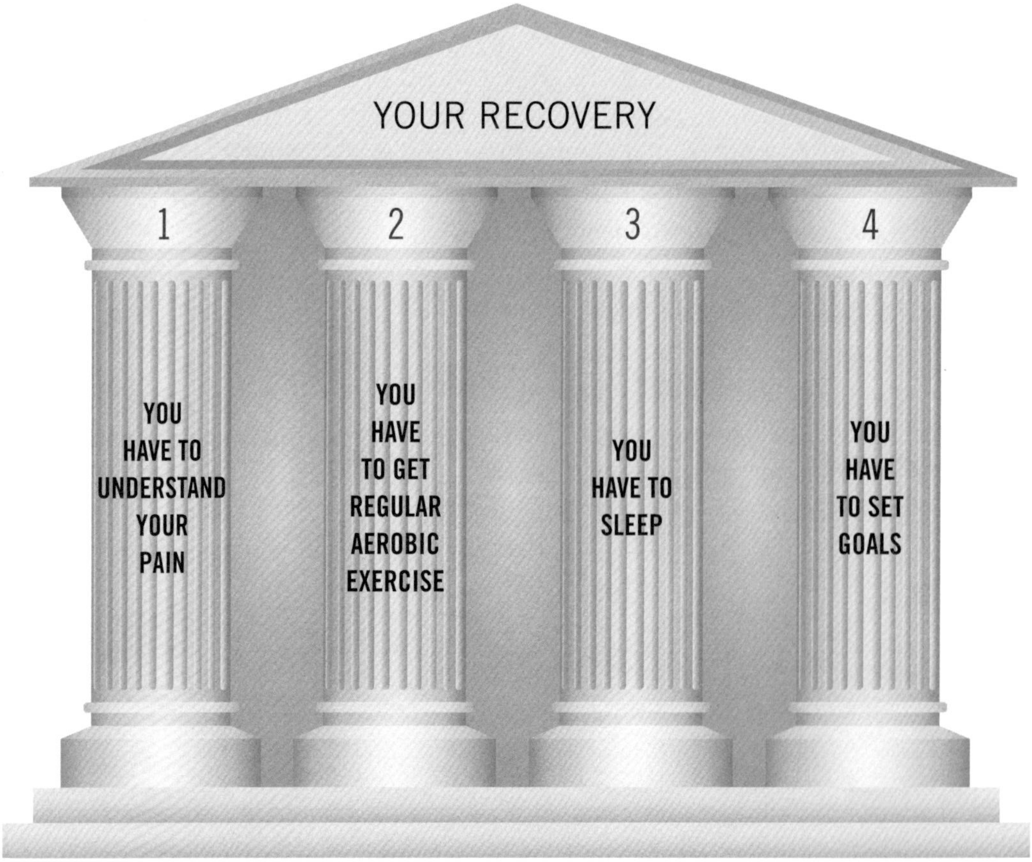

1. **Pain education**

Want some really good news? You're well on your way with this one. Education is treatment.[7,8] Gaining an understanding of the neuroscience of your pain will ease some of your fears, explain unknowns and provide hope. This alone will move you forward to recovery. Studies have shown that your nerves will steadily calm down the more you learn about pain. This is a sophisticated alarm system, and if you have been struggling for a prolonged period, it will only turn down a little bit at a time.[10] Read your workbook; go through it again and again. Write down questions and ask your healthcare provider.

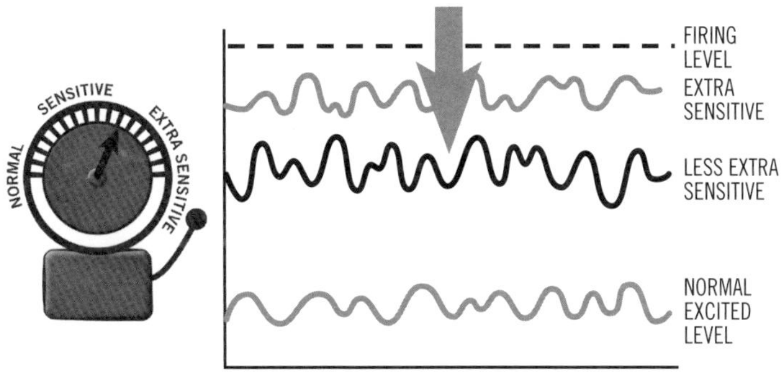

2. **Aerobic exercise**

Research has shown that aerobic exercise, which gets your heart pumping a little faster and pumps blood and oxygen through your body, helps calm nerves down.[28] Don't worry, you don't need to run marathons or climb mountains (though eventually you could if you wanted to!). There is a definite time and intensity needed in aerobic exercise to ease pain. Without getting too complicated or scientific, the average person with pain will need to do aerobic exercise for just over 10 minutes and get their heart rate up around 100-110 beats per minute to receive benefit.[29] This can be a brisk walk, light jog, biking, aerobics, swimming and more.

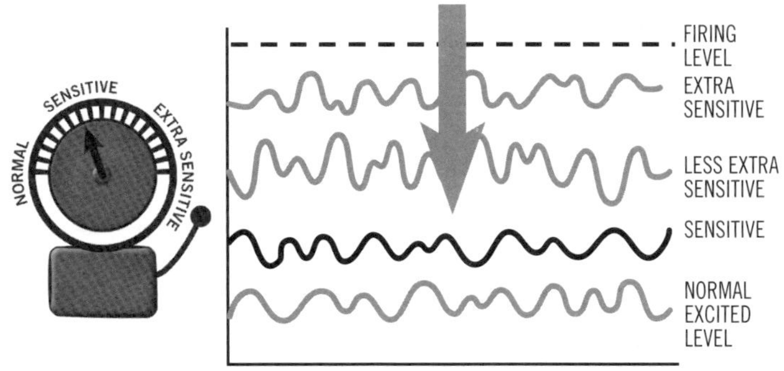

Also, remember that if you pump blood and oxygen through your body regularly, you will achieve additional benefits:

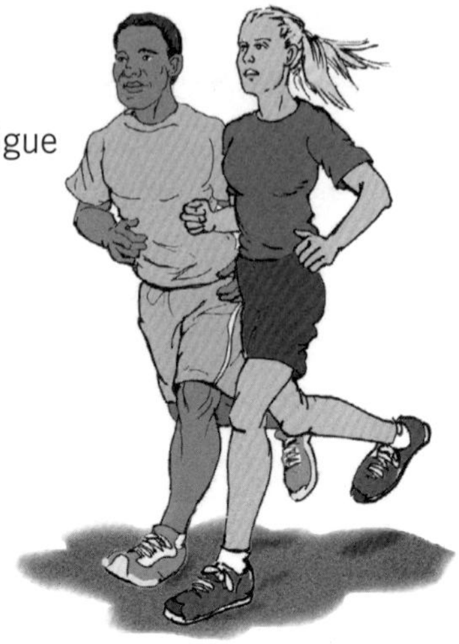

- ✔ Better sleep
- ✔ Weight loss
- ✔ Decreased stress levels
- ✔ Less muscle soreness and fatigue
- ✔ Fewer mood swings
- ✔ Decreased or no depression

When it comes to exercise and pain, we often see two mistakes. First, some people do "too much" and believe "more is better" (no pain, no gain). This is not the case. If you ignore pain, it will increase. On the flipside, if you do very little or nothing, pain will also increase (if it hurts, don't do it).

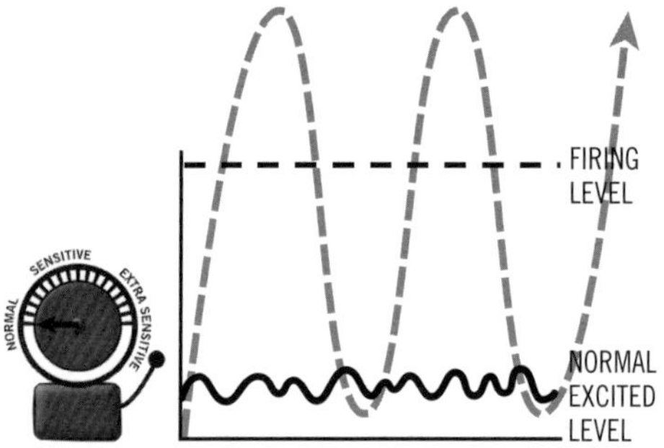

"No pain, no gain"

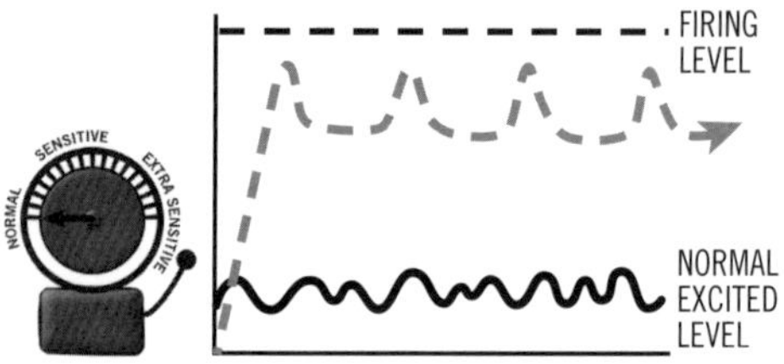

"If it hurts, don't do it"

The answer is to start easy and build slowly.[6] Studies have shown that by starting with only three minutes of walking and then adding one minute every other day, you can progress over time to healthy regular exercise.[30] Also, remember that if you "feel" your back, leg or arm during exercise, it's just your sensitive nervous system telling you you're exercising, rather than something being wrong.

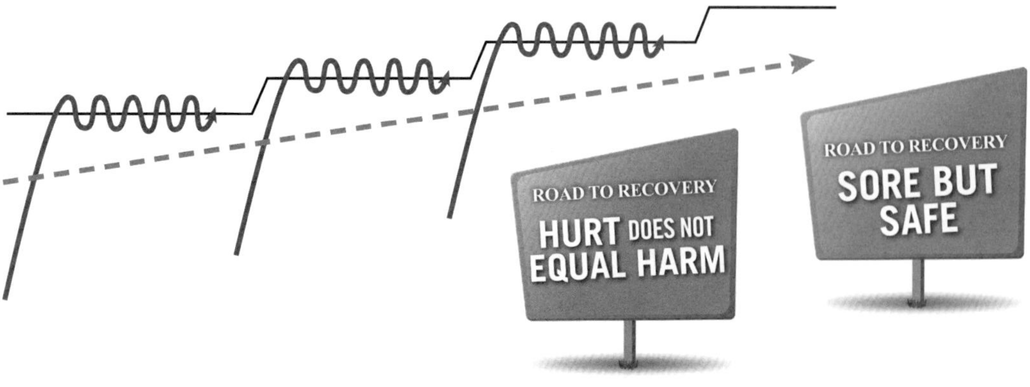

Your aerobic exercise plan

Research shows that 90% of exercise is setting up a plan, so let's set one up:

☐ **MEASURE YOUR CURRENT RESTING HEART RATE:** Find your pulse on your wrist or neck, and count the beats for 10 seconds. Multiply by six. Your resting heart rate is:________. Remember that you only need to get your heart rate up to 100-110 beats/minute, so it won't take much to get it there.

☐ **CHOOSE YOUR EXERCISE:** Make it something easily accessible, such as walking. If walking is not an option, substitute with biking or swimming.

☐ Walking ☐ Biking ☐ Swimming ☐ Other:________________

☐ **CHOOSE THE DAYS OF THE WEEK YOU'LL BE DOING THE EXERCISE:** We suggest five days a week, with two days off. Best to schedule a few days of exercise, a rest day, a few more days of exercise and then a day off. Schedule around your work, daily activities and family tasks to avoid undue stress.

SUN.	MON.	TUES.	WED.	THURS.	FRI.	SAT.
☐	☐	☐	☐	☐	☐	☐

☐ **PICK A TIME OF DAY YOU'LL DO THE EXERCISE:** The time can be different on different days. Write the time you will exercise next to the days checked above.

☐ **LET PEOPLE KNOW YOUR PLAN:** You can share this with a spouse, a friend, a work colleague or a family member. Better yet, ask them to join you!

☐ **START SMALL:** If you have not done much exercise lately, do as little as three to five minutes to get started. Remember, you are very sore and sensitive. Take it slow, but get going. Every two to three days, add a minute. The goal is to reach 20-30 minutes of exercise, five days a week.

☐ **LOG YOUR PROGRESS:** Write down the day, date, time, duration and something positive that happened in your day. Log your sleep hours as well.

3. Sleep hygiene

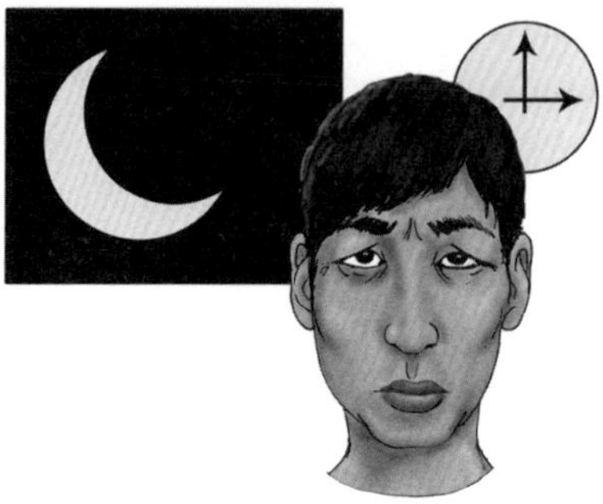

Few things have as huge of an effect on our health as sleep. At least eight hours of sleep is needed for most people. Americans average six hours a night and people in pain average less. Even if you sleep a lot, you never feel refreshed when you wake. Sleep deprivation has been linked to increased rates of pain, obesity, depression and other health-related disorders. Changing sleep habits takes work, but is important for your recovery. The following sleep hygiene program comes from the best sleep centers in the world. As with exercise, start easy and build slowly. For example, look at the list and pick the easiest one you can do tonight. Tomorrow night repeat that task and add another. Every few days, add another one. If you're the classic person struggling to sleep at night and typically fall asleep at 3am in front of the TV, it may be hard to start going to bed at 10pm. So, every day, go to bed 15 minutes earlier, until you reach the desired goal. These small steps are not as hard on your system.

Your sleep hygiene program

- ☐ Set a time to go to bed
- ☐ Quiet the house by turning off the computer and TV one hour before you plan to go to sleep
- ☐ Reduce fluid intake in the evening
- ☐ Reduce alcoholic beverages in the late evening
- ☐ Darken and cool the bedroom
- ☐ Remove kids and pets from your bed
- ☐ Eliminate daytime naps; if naps are needed, limit them to power naps of less than 20 minutes
- ☐ Exercise during the day
- ☐ Park your ideas; place a notepad and pen next to your bed
- ☐ Relax, meditate or read a book before bed
- ☐ Avoid checking emails or messages before bed
- ☐ Stay in bed...if you cannot sleep, close your eyes and relax
- ☐ Set a wake time, and stay in bed until then
- ☐ Avoid caffeine in the late afternoons or evenings

4. Goal setting

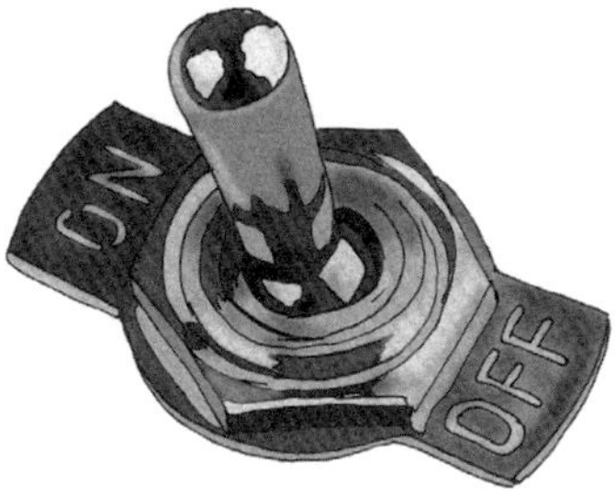

The final pillar of your program is setting goals.[11] Yes, while you hurt, thinking about goals is very hard. The motivation part of your brain is constantly in pain meetings and the lion is draining all your energy. But having specific goals is crucial to this process. As a means to set goals, we're going to do a little task: Imagine there's an "on-off" switch on your back. If we could reach behind your back, turn the switch "off" and instantly get rid of all your pain, or ease it so much you're not even that aware of it, what would you do again? What things that you used to do before pain would you do again?

Make a list. Pick the top three things you'd love to do again, if pain was not around:

1.____

2.____

3.____

Now that you have three things you'd like to do again, pick your top one:

____

For your top goal, find some smaller steps. Everything in life can be broken down into smaller pieces.

- For example, dinner can be prepared during the course of a day or even days. Ingredients can be prepared and stored. This decreases standing for long periods of time, resulting in a fun time cooking, with little to no pain.
- Not all laundry has to be washed, folded or pressed in one shot.
- Not all emails have to be answered at one time. Set a number, perhaps three to four every hour, thus limiting sitting for long periods.
- A party can be planned, prepared for and executed in small steps.

What else can turn the pharmacy on?

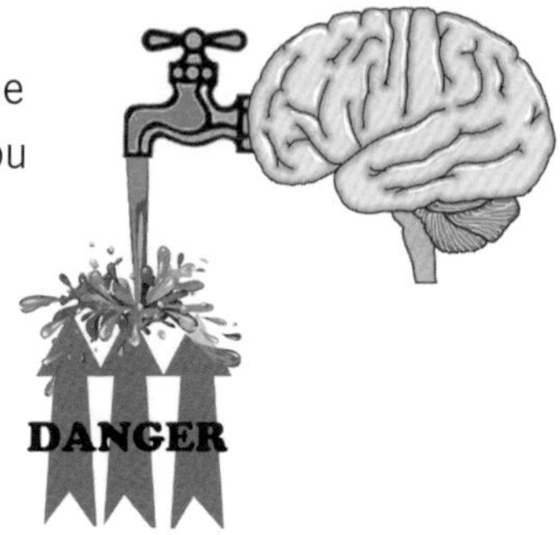

As we said before, there are many different ways to get the brain producing pain medicine again without drugs. As you look at the list of treatments that have shown to turn a dry brain into a wet brain, you will notice some that you have tried. If they worked, you would not be going through this workbook, right? Why didn't they work? The easy answer is that pain is complex and many bodily systems are involved. On their own, none of these treatments (including the four pillars) are that powerful. When several of these are combined, and (more importantly) the four pillars form the cornerstone of your recovery, you are more likely to succeed.

- ✔ Relaxation
- ✔ Aquatic therapy
- ✔ Nerve glides
- ✔ Breathing exercises
- ✔ Humor
- ✔ Journaling
- ✔ Yoga
- ✔ General conditioning
- ✔ Social interaction
- ✔ Meditation and mindfulness
- ✔ Massage
- ✔ Diet
- ✔ Modalities
- ✔ Trigger point therapy
- ✔ Medication
- ✔ Spirituality
- ✔ Manual therapy
- ✔ Coping skills

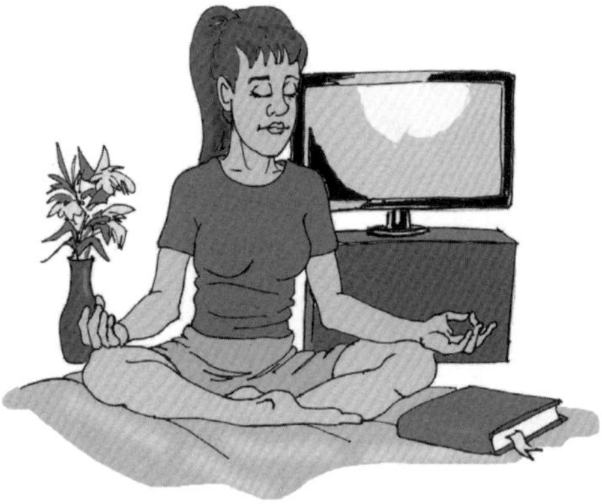

You will notice there are many other strategies, but once again: The four pillars have to be in place. This workbook focuses heavily on the four pillars. We suggest that you and your healthcare provider discuss this list and, upon setting the four pillars in place, chose additional treatments, if needed. They should coincide with your interest, the provider's skill set and your overall path to recovery.

TASK 7

As you look at the four pillars for recovery, which one(s) do you think will pose the biggest challenge? What barriers exist? What can you do to overcome these barriers?

If "fixing" pain was easy, this workbook would not be needed. If "fixing" pain was easy, all the treatments you have received should have worked. If "fixing" pain is easy, then why are we spending billions of dollars on pain treatments and why are pain numbers getting worse, not better? Pain is complex, but it doesn't need to be. The material covered in this book is based off the most advanced pain science, but rather than focusing on one single issue, it looks at the broader perspective of pain. In studies where we track people going through this program one year later and even years later, pain eases considerably and even goes away.[31,32] As pain eases and you do more, you will reclaim your life. Steadily, over time, you will notice yourself doing more and more, while being less aware and bothered by your pain. The ultimate goal is to understand pain so well, you become less afraid of it and, despite the pain, get on with your life.[11,33]

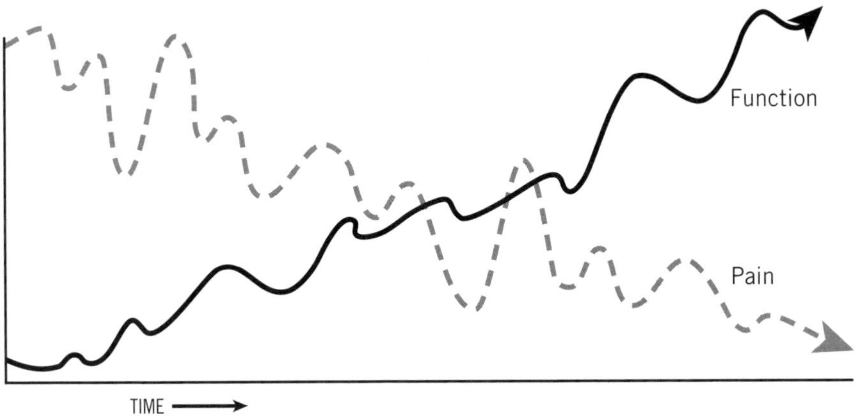

You will notice from the graph above the path has ups and downs. Nerves and their sensitivity, and ultimately your pain, is a barometer for the stresses in your life and has (just like us), good and bad days. Don't get discouraged when you have a "flare-up." This is quite normal and may indicate a response to some stress at work or home, or perhaps you did a little too much activity and need to back off a little. Stay the course. Keep with the program. The program works. It's hard work and is 100 percent up to you to make it work, but it works.

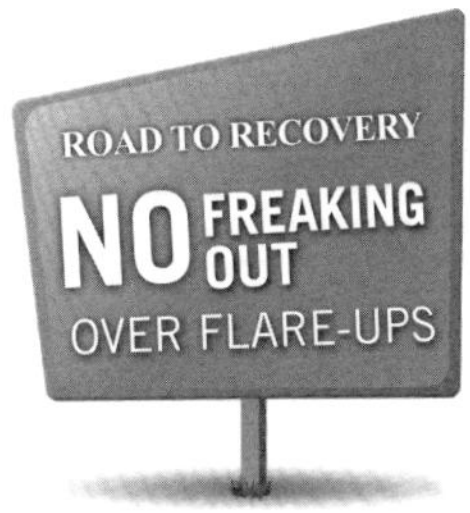

We're hoping you can see there is light at the end of the tunnel. You can get better. This workbook is based on dozens of studies we have conducted and thousands of patients. We have seen that it IS possible: You can take control of your pain and stop pain from controlling what you can and cannot do. We hope many of the issues we have dealt with in this workbook have helped you, in essence, paint your yellow flags green, as you can see on your workbook's cover. By getting a handle on these issues, the threat is steadily reduced, and guess what? The alarm system and your pain eases.

It is time to leave the roundabout. Yes, unbeknownst to many Americans, you CAN leave a roundabout! The various steps we outlined in this workbook, along with the guidance and help from a healthcare professional familiar with this work, can get you back to a fulfilling, meaningful life that is not controlled by pain.

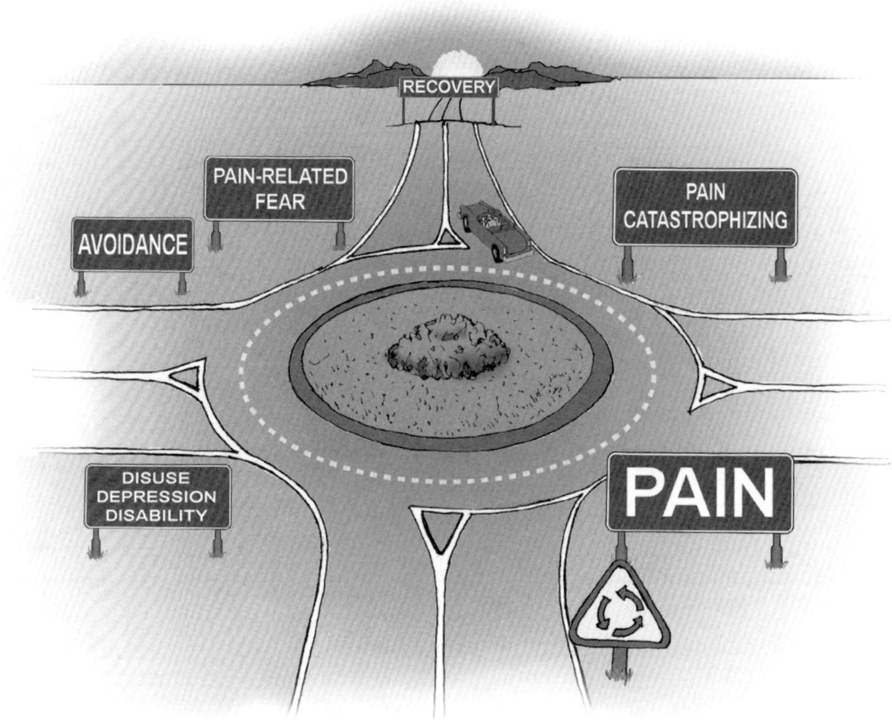

TASK 8

The graph on page 33 shows that as your pain is calming down, your function will come up. Many people believe they shouldn't or can't function better until all of their pain is gone, but in reality, getting more active actually helps the pain to decrease. They happen simultaneously. How ready do you feel to press forward with your program, even though you will likely continue to have some pain as you start?

Scientific support for your recovery

1. Moseley GL. Reconceptualising pain according to modern pain sciences. *Physical Therapy Reviews.* 2007;12:169-178.
2. Nijs J, Roussel N, Paul van Wilgen C, Koke A, Smeets R. Thinking beyond muscles and joints: therapists' and patients' attitudes and beliefs regarding chronic musculoskeletal pain are key to applying effective treatment. *Manual Therapy.* Apr 2013;18(2):96-102.
3. Melzack R. Pain and the neuromatrix in the brain Journal of Dental Education. 2001;65:1378-1382.
4. Gifford LS. Pain, the tissues and the nervous system. *Physiotherapy.* 1998;84:27-33.
5. Louw A, Butler DS, Diener I, Puentedura EJ. Development of a preoperative neuroscience educational program for patients with lumbar radiculopathy. *American Journal of Physical Medicine & Rehabilitation/Association of Academic Physiatrists.* May 2013;92(5):446-452.
6. Gifford L. *Aches and Pains.* Cornwall: Wordpress; 2014.
7. Louw A, Diener I, Butler DS, Puentedura EJ. The effect of neuroscience education on pain, disability, anxiety, and stress in chronic musculoskeletal pain. *Archives of Physical Medicine and Rehabilitation.* Dec 2011;92(12):2041-2056.
8. Louw A, Zimney K, Puentedura EJ, Diener I. The efficacy of pain neuroscience education on musculoskeletal pain: A systematic review of the literature. *Physiotherapy Theory and Practice.* Jul 2016;32(5):332-355.
9. Moseley GL. Unravelling the barriers to reconceptualisation of the problem in chronic pain: the actual and perceived ability of patients and health professionals to understand the neurophysiology. *Journal of Pain.* 2003;4(4):184-189.
10. Nijs J, Paul van Wilgen C, Van Oosterwijck J, van Ittersum M, Meeus M. How to explain central sensitization to patients with 'unexplained' chronic musculoskeletal pain: practice guidelines. *Manual Therapy.* Oct 2011;16(5):413-418.
11. Louw A, Zimney K, O'Hotto C, Hilton S. The clinical application of teaching people about pain. *Physiotherapy Theory and Practice.* Jul 2016;32(5):385-395.
12. Vlaeyen JWS, Linton SJ. Fear-avoidance and its consequences in chronic musculoskeletal pain: a state of the art. *Pain.* 2000;85:317-322.
13. Louw A. *Why Do I Hurt? A Neuroscience Approach to Pain.* Minneapolis: OPTP; 2013.
14. Nahin RL. Estimates of pain prevalence and severity in adults: United States, 2012. *The Journal of Pain: Official Journal of the American Pain Society.* Aug 2015;16(8):769-780.
15. Kendall NAS, Linton SJ, Main CJ. *Guide to assessing psychosocial yellow flags in acute low back pain: risk factors for long term disability and work loss.* Wellington: Accident Rehabilitation & Compensation Insurance Corporation of New Zealand and the National Health Committee; 1997.
16. Okada E, Matsumoto M, Ichihara D, et al. Aging of the cervical spine in healthy volunteers: a 10-year longitudinal magnetic resonance imaging study. *Spine.* Apr 1 2009;34(7):706-712.
17. Simotas AC, Shen T. Neck pain in demolition derby drivers. *Archives of Physical Medicine and Rehabilitation.* Apr 2005;86(4):693-696.
18. Spielmann AL, Forster BB, Kokan P, Hawkins RH, Janzen DL. Shoulder after rotator cuff repair: MR imaging findings in asymptomatic individuals--initial experience. *Radiology.* Dec 1999;213(3):705-708.
19. Reilly P, Macleod I, Macfarlane R, Windley J, Emery RJ. Dead men and radiologists don't lie: a review of cadaveric and radiological studies of rotator cuff tear prevalence. *Annals of the Royal College of Surgeons of England.* Mar 2006;88(2):116-121.
20. Kjaer P, Leboeuf-Yde C, Korsholm L, Sorensen JS, Bendix T. Magnetic resonance imaging and low back pain in adults: a diagnostic imaging study of 40-year-old men and women. *Spine.* May 15 2005;30(10):1173-1180.
21. Twomey LT, Taylor JR. Age changes in lumbar vertebrae and intervertebral discs. *Clinical Orthopaedics and Related Research.* Nov 1987(224):97-104.
22. Register B, Pennock AT, Ho CP, Strickland CD, Lawand A, Philippon MJ. Prevalence of abnormal hip findings in asymptomatic participants: a prospective, blinded study. *American Journal of Sports Medicine.* Dec 2012;40(12):2720-2724.
23. Silvis ML, Mosher TJ, Smetana BS, et al. High prevalence of pelvic and hip magnetic resonance imaging findings in asymptomatic collegiate and professional hockey players. *American Journal of Sports Medicine.* Apr 2011;39(4):715-721.
24. Munk B, Lundorf E, Jensen J. Long-term outcome of meniscal degeneration in the knee: poor association between MRI and symptoms in 45 patients followed more than 4 years. *Acta Orthopaedica Scandinavica.* Feb 2004;75(1):89-92.
25. Major NM, Helms CA. MR imaging of the knee: findings in asymptomatic collegiate basketball players. *American Journal of Roentgenology.* Sep 2002;179(3):641-644.
26. Puentedura EJ, Louw A. A neuroscience approach to managing athletes with low back pain. *Physical Therapy in Sport.* Aug 2012;13(3):123-133.
27. Sapolsky R. *Why Zebras Don't Get Ulcers.* New York: W.H. Freeman and Company 1994.
28. Kuphal KE, Fibuch EE, Taylor BK. Extended swimming exercise reduces inflammatory and peripheral neuropathic pain in rodents. *Journal of Pain.* Dec 2007;8(12):989-997.
29. Hoffman MD, Shepanski MA, Mackenzie SP, Clifford PS. Experimentally induced pain perception is acutely reduced by aerobic exercise in people with chronic low back pain. *Journal of Rehabilitation Research and Development.* Mar-Apr 2005;42(2):183-190.
30. Fulcher KY, White PD. Randomised controlled trial of graded exercise in patients with the chronic fatigue syndrome. *British Medical Journal.* Jun 7 1997;314(7095):1647-1652.
31. Moseley L. Combined physiotherapy and education is efficacious for chronic low back pain. *Australian Journal of Physiotherapy.* 2002;48(4):297-302.
32. Louw A, Diener I, Landers MR, Puentedura EJ. Preoperative Pain Neuroscience Education for Lumbar Radiculopathy: A Multicenter Randomized Controlled Trial With 1-Year Follow-up. *Spine.* Aug 15 2014;39(18):1449-1457.
33. Louw A, Puentedura EJ, Zimney K, Schmidt S. Know Pain, Know Gain? A Perspective on Pain Neuroscience Education in Physical Therapy. *The Journal of Orthopaedic and Sports Physical Therapy.* Mar 2016;46(3):131-134.

More patient books by Adriaan Louw

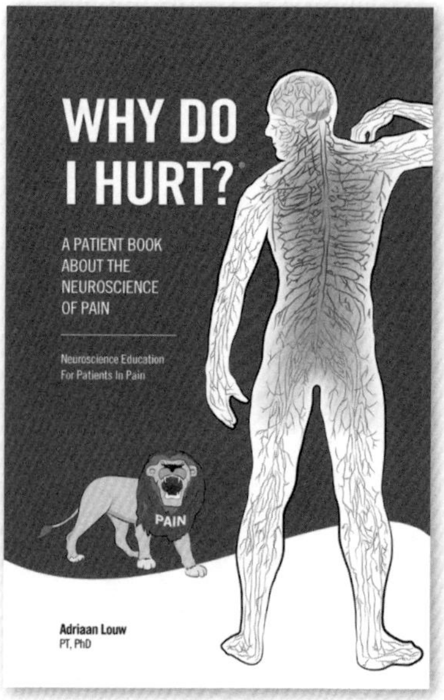

Why Do I Hurt?
A Patient Book About the Neuroscience of Pain
ITEM #8746

Why Do I Hurt?
teaches about the science of pain in simple language using metaphors, examples and images, followed by treatment strategies to help you start feeling better.

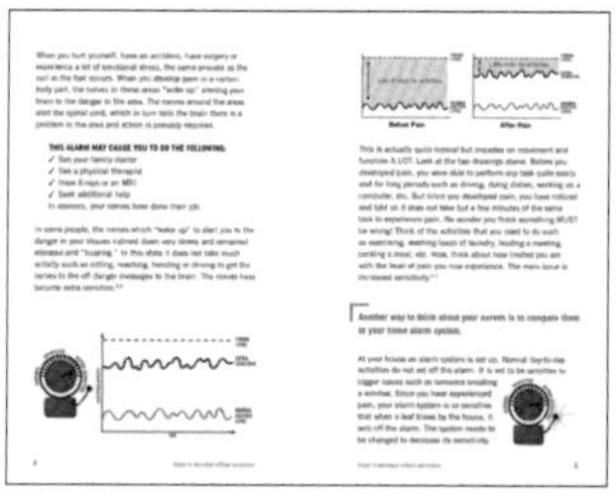

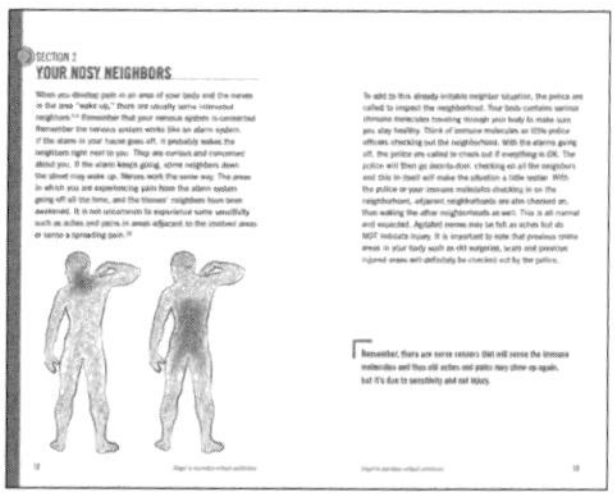

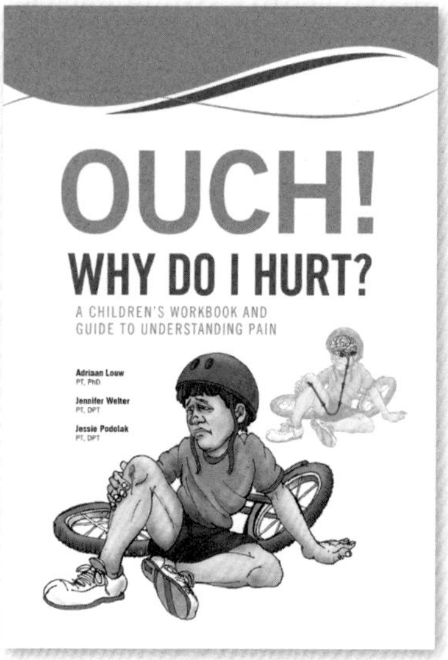

Ouch! Why Do I Hurt?
A Children's Workbook and Guide to Understanding Pain
ITEM# 8755

This workbook and guide provides a fun, interactive way to teach kids about how pain works and what to do about it. Written in simple, easy-to-understand language, the book uses colorful illustrations and activities to help teach kids about the body's amazing protective system—the nervous system. It then provides healthy ways for kids to manage pain when they experience it.

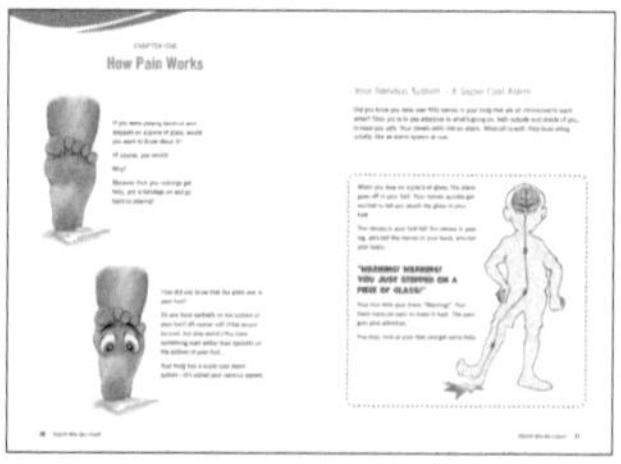

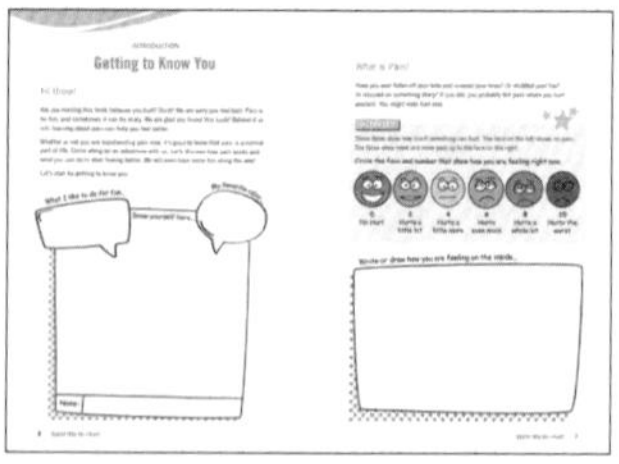

Adriaan Louw's patient books and clinical resources are available exclusively from OPTP.
OPTP.com I 800.367.7393

More patient books by Adriaan Louw

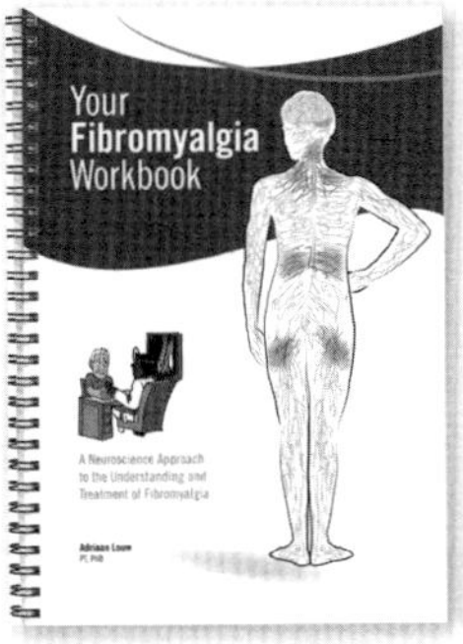

Your Fibromyalgia Workbook
ITEM# 8747

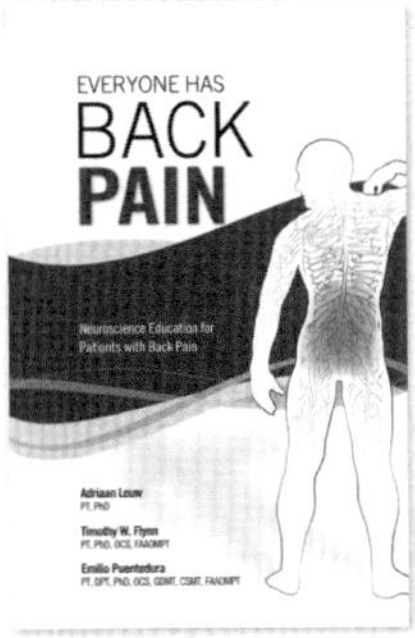

Everyone Has Back Pain
ITEM #8754

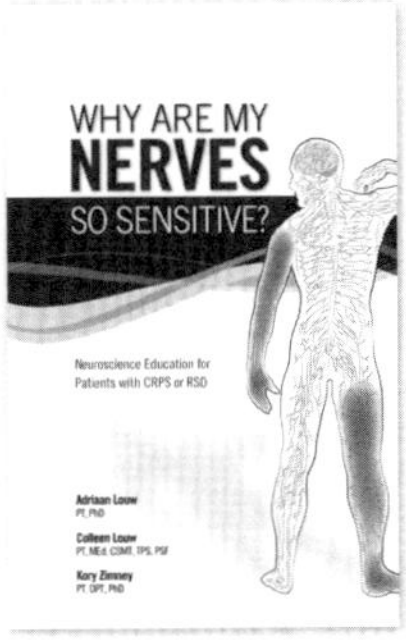

Why Are My Nerves So Sensitive?
ITEM #8752

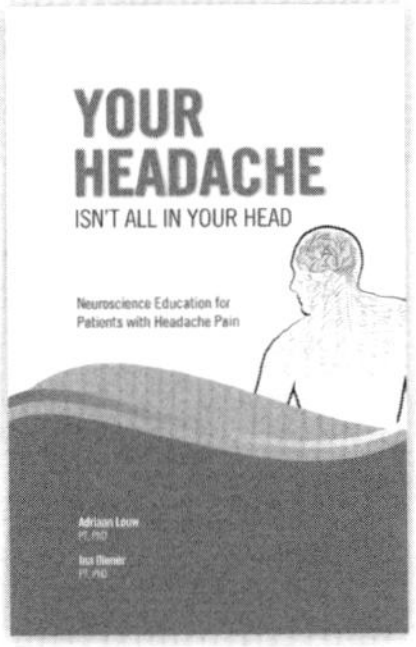

Your Headache Isn't All In Your Head
ITEM #8749

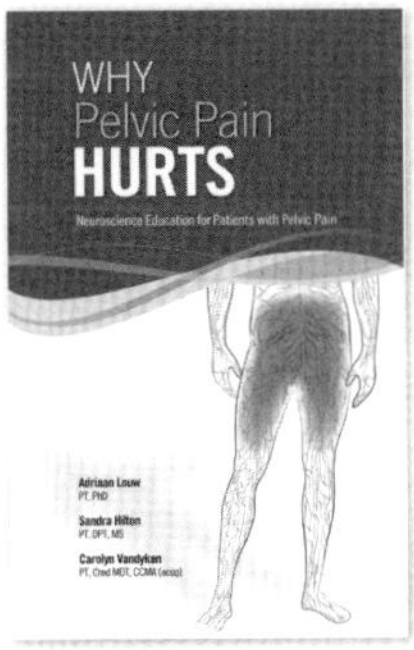

Why Pelvic Pain Hurts
ITEM #8742

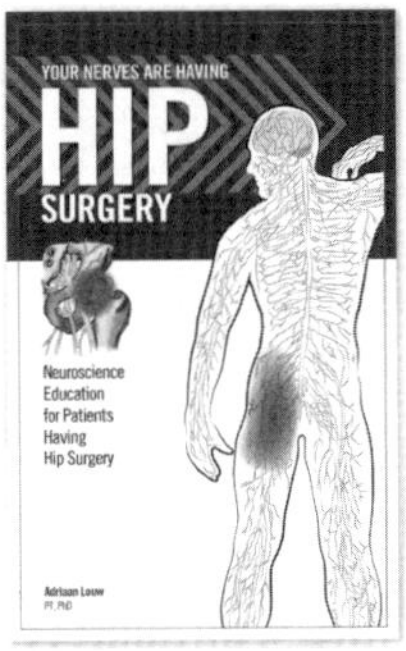

Your Nerves Are Having Hip Surgery
ITEM #8757

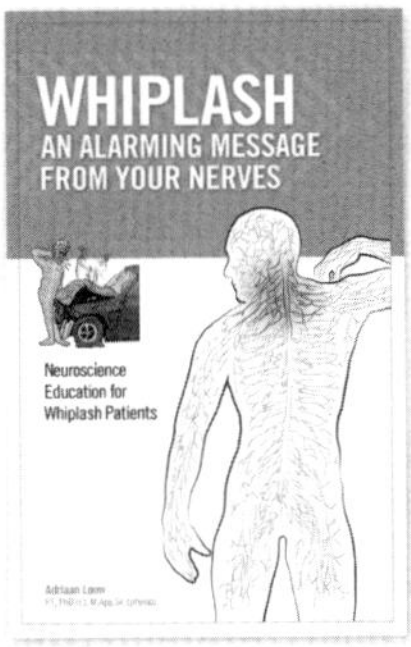

Whiplash: An Alarming Message from Your Nerves
ITEM #8744

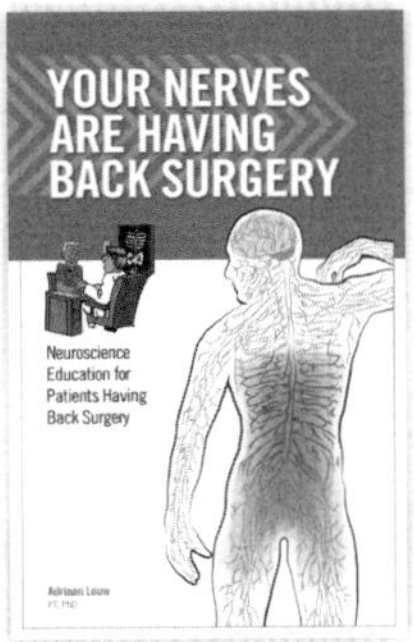

Your Nerves Are Having Back Surgery
ITEM #8745

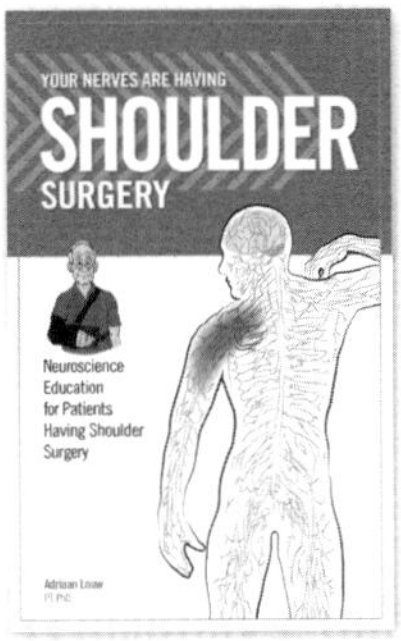

Your Nerves Are Having Shoulder Surgery
ITEM #8750

Clinical resources by Adriaan Louw

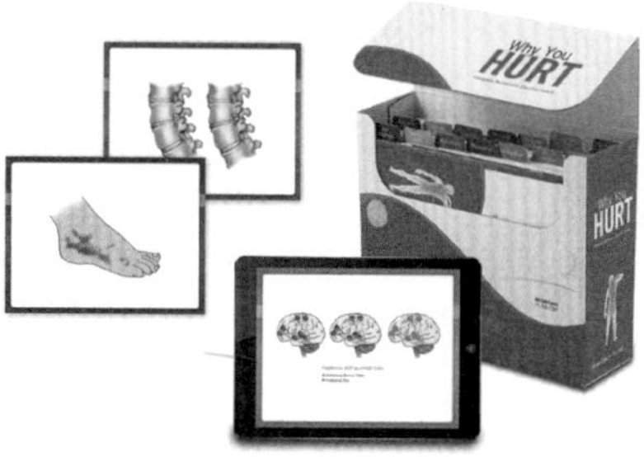

Why You Hurt: Pain Neuroscience Education System
ITEM #8751

This all-inclusive system is an interactive tool that will help you engage in meaningful discussions with your patients and teach them what pain really is and how it works. It contains education cards, teaching cues, homework cards and more.

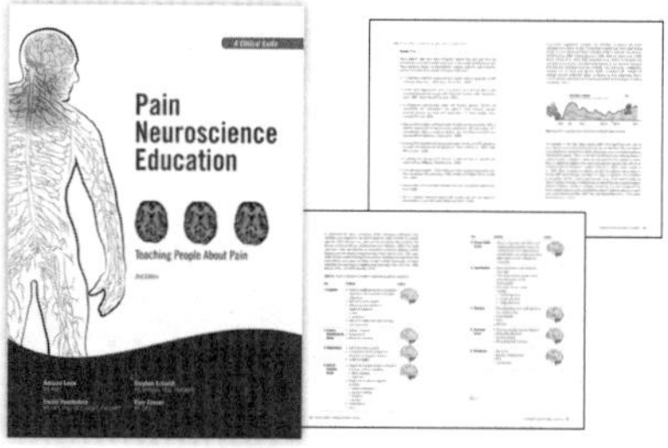

Pain Neuroscience Education: Teaching People About Pain
ITEM #8748-2

Written by clinicians for clinicians,this 536-page textbook delivers an evidence-based perspective on how the body and brain work together to create pain and shows how to teach and convey this new view of pain to patients in a way that's easy to understand.

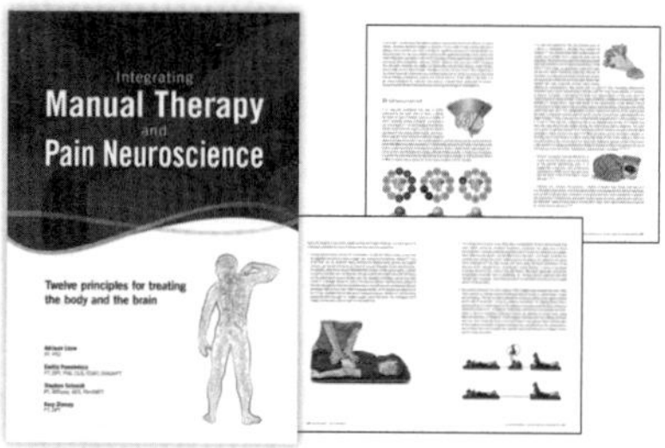

Integrating Manual Therapy and Pain Neuroscience
ITEM #8758

This 272-page text uses 12 principles of treatment to show how the integration of manual therapy and pain science can help clinicians provide better treatment and improve patient outcomes.

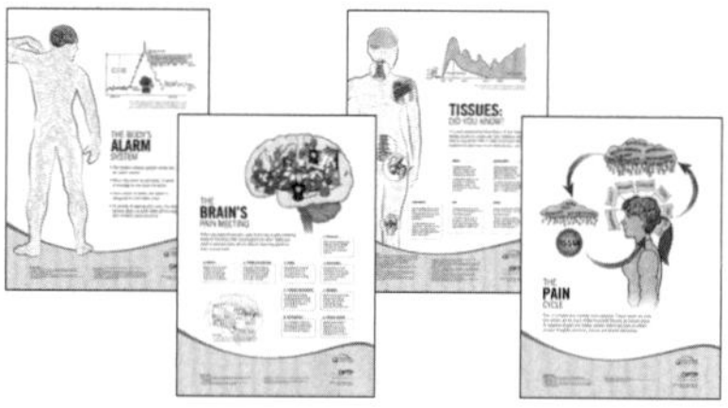

Pain Neuroscience Education Posters
ITEM #876SET

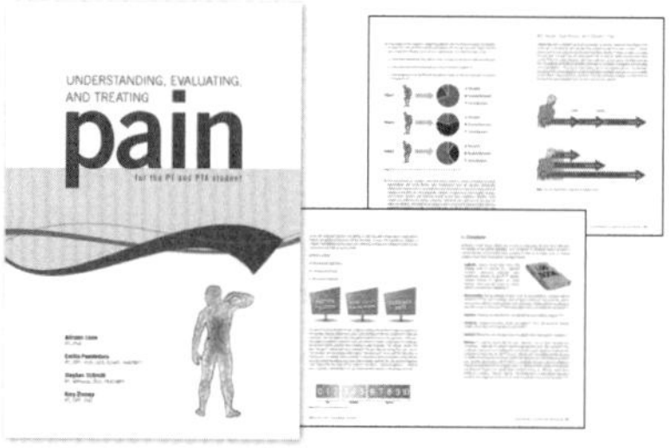

Understanding, Evaluating, and Treating Pain for the PT and PTA Student
ITEM #8759

Based on current guidelines for PT school curriculums, this 224-page clinical guide provides a foundation for PT and PTA students to learn about pain and provides the tools to help them be part of the solution to this global epidemic.

Adriaan Louw's patient books and clinical resources are available exclusively from OPTP.
OPTP.com I 800.367.7393